LONGEVITY
SECRETS

An Anti-aging Guide to Preventing Disease, Staying
Active, Avoiding Memory Loss, and Living Longer

Tammy Gallagher, FNLP

www.tamgall.com

and complete information. No warranties of any kind are declared or implied. Readers acknowledge that the author is not rendering legal, financial, medical, or any other professional advice. The content within this book has been derived from various sources. Please consult a licensed professional before attempting any techniques outlined in this book.

The use of this information is at the readers' own risk. By reading this document, the reader agrees that under no circumstances is the author responsible for any direct or indirect losses incurred because of the use of the information contained within this document, including, but not limited to, — errors, omissions, or inaccuracies.

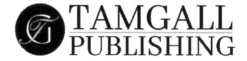

CONTENTS

Just for You!

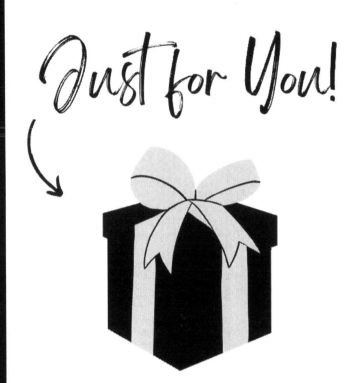

A FREE GIFT FOR OUR READERS

Get my free eBook on sweeteners...the good, the bad and the ugly. Which sweeteners to avoid and which provide health benefits.

Visit *www.tamgall.com/sweeteners-ebook*

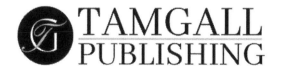

TAMGALL
PUBLISHING

INTRODUCTION

If you had a chance to choose, would you wish to live past 100 years? The desire to live longer is an innate wish in all humans. And rightfully so. The body can naturally wade off illnesses and protect us from danger. Then why do some people live to their 60's while others live past 100? Why is it that seemingly healthy people die from disease?

Aging is a complex process. Our body cells are programmed to self-renew to pave the way for healthier cells. But often, the foods we eat and our environment trigger harmful substances that speed up aging. It is no surprise that even with the advances in health advocacy programs, many people are affected by chronic illnesses, such as hypertension, type two diabetes, kidney disease, dementia, autoimmune, and mental disorders. These diseases result in lifelong dependence on medication and can cause severe repercussions such as neuropathy.

Chronic illness causes physical pain and stress and interferes with the quality of life. As these issues develop, medication is costly, affecting family finances and significantly reducing living pleasure. Those affected suffer from pain and lose the freedom to enjoy life without good health. I have good news for you. Implementing the strategies I share can increase your odds of preventing most of these diseases.

What if being old does not equate to getting lifestyle diseases?

Longevity is influenced by gene expression and how our genes respond to environmental factors. You can prevent most chronic illnesses and improve your quality of life with the proper diet and lifestyle interventions. You will not need to deal with the long-term consequences of such diseases.

Is it possible to live to 100 without suffering from chronic diseases? Prevention is the only solution to save the cost of health care, improve the quality of life, and enjoy getting older. Although being healthy does not mean you will always be free from disease, some interventions can give you a healthy old age and fulfilling life.

Recently, there has been an upsurge in cosmetic products and procedures that promise to revitalize aging skin. However, longevity must be approached from all angles through diet, lifestyle, and managing stress and emotions. There is no magic pill. It is about giving the body the capacity to heal itself from the factors that cause illness.

This book shares how the five pillars of a longer life, such as nutrition, exercise, sleep, gut health, and stress management, can influence your health. It provides well-researched and time-tested ideologies for longevity. The goal is not only to extend your time but also to improve your living pleasure. I have more good news. You can accomplish this with interventions that promote well-being and reduce stress, such as meditation, exercise, and healthy sleeping patterns.

This book seeks to enlighten you about your body's healing power and how you can enhance it through the five pillars. It is the only manual you will need on how to live a long healthy life no matter your health condition. You will learn how to implement the pillars of longevity that you can use to protect your body before disease strikes. You will also learn to be active and happy even if you already have a chronic illness requiring long-term attention. Indeed, you can reverse chronic inflammation and disease effects and change your lifestyle to enhance your quality of life.

You will learn how to attain optimum health and longevity through a holistic approach that considers all physical and emotional health aspects. Taking care of these aspects of your health will give you more vitality, improve your memory, prevent disease, make you feel and look younger, and have a happy and active life. You will take stock of current habits affecting your health and implement a sustainable health plan to increase your energy, better your immunity, get better sleep, reduce illness, improve your memory, and have less stress.

Longevity Secrets will give you a multi-tier approach focusing on prevention aspects like nutrition and lifestyle within your control. In each chapter, you will get practical strategies for practicing each pillar.

Change is a gradual process marred by obstacles along the way. The concluding chapter will bring it all together in a step-by-step plan of action and show you how to apply the longevity secrets one at a time, integrate what you learned into your life, and forge a path of longevity.

Cultivating new healthy habits takes time. It takes about twenty-one days (around three weeks) to ingrain a new habit. This book will guide you on how to implement longevity secrets sustainably and be healthy from the inside out. The repetitions make the brain get used to it and become second nature. Repetition is the mother of skill. The habits will transform and rejuvenate your life. When you build better habits and commit to longevity secrets, you will achieve all that and more. The power is in your hands.

Where All This Began

My interest in longevity is a story of personal empowerment to get over my struggles with health. I was obese in my 20s and struggled with my weight for the better part of my adult life. And because misery loves company, that brought in the other cocktail of lifestyle diseases. I had high blood pressure and high cholesterol, and developed Crohn's disease in 2011.

I would say developing Crohn's disease was a blessing in disguise, but I wouldn't wish it on anyone. You must not wait to experience disease before you decide to become healthy. Some diseases cannot be reversed, but they can be prevented.

In the quest to improve my life and keep off these trails of illnesses that were interfering with my life, I sought to improve my health. I discovered that what I ate, combined with physical activity, among other factors, was the key to slowing down the aging process and regaining my health.

I went back to college in my 50s to pursue nutrition to learn how to live a healthy life despite my previous health challenges. Through my own experience and getting accredited in functional nutrition and lifestyle, I have assisted many people since 2018 going through similar issues through my clinic, Ballantyne Weight Loss Center. The easiest way to help others lose weight is to get the body in balance, and that means dealing with a wide range of disease and illness. Only then will diet and lifestyle modifications be achievable.

I used my knowledge to get my health back. I lost 78 pounds and slowed down the aging process, making me younger than my years. I desire to help you lead a healthier and more active life, just as I have done for myself and my patients. Through my pain, I want to alleviate your suffering and help you love your life so much that getting older will not be a source of alarm but a sense of pride in the healthy life you built for yourself. My achievement of attaining the healthiest version of myself is an invitation to everyone who struggles with weight and does not know if they will ever be free of pain.

You can control your future; your lifestyle is the key to a healthier and longer life. You do not have to wait until it is too late before you change your habits. Prevention is the solution to avoiding chronic pain in old age due to chronic illness. You do not have to spend much on costly medication or procedures. You can take these steps now into your healthiest future. And no, it will not take one day or a week to change. Changing from unhealthy habits takes time. It took me ten years to get to where I am. But one step at a time, you will make the transition manageable and enjoyable, and sustainable health you will enjoy for the rest of your life.

Are you ready to learn about the five pillars of longevity and how you can become healthier today? Keep reading...

1

FIVE PILLARS OF LONGEVITY

Longevity Secrets explores the five pillars of good health and unlocks the secrets of healthy aging. These pillars must occur in your life for a healthy body and mind and to add healthy years to your life. I have helped many improve their lives and guided them to take charge through nutrition and lifestyle modifications, and I will help you discover what is possible too.

The first pillar is sleep, which is non-negotiable for a long, healthy life. I will address why getting no less than seven hours of natural sleep every night is crucial and how you can improve your quality and quantity of sleep. Sleep deprivation is associated with adverse health outcomes such as impaired immune function, increased risk of type two diabetes, cardiovascular disease, obesity, depression, and accidents from drowsy driving.[1] Furthermore, it helps you manage a healthy weight by reducing your appetite. After reading this chapter, you will never treat sleep as a luxury but as a necessary tool to improve your memory, keep you alert, perform better at work, and prevent diseases.

You will see how nutrition is vital for keeping you alive and healthy. You will learn to adopt the philosophy of eating to live, not living to eat, if longevity is your goal. A healthy eating plan helps achieve and maintain a healthy weight, supports the muscles, bones, and digestive system, and lowers the risk of diseases such as type two diabetes, cardiovascular diseases, and some cancers.

The Mediterranean Diet is the gold standard for a healthy and long life. It promotes the intake of whole grains, seafood, fruits, vegetables, healthy fats, and wine. I'll also introduce the MMD, my personal modified Mediterranean Diet if you want to take your nutrition to longevity extremes.

You will discover that it's not only what you eat, but how and when you eat also counts. You will learn how to use intermittent fasting to control food intake, optimize metabolism, and boost cell regeneration. Yes, you can stimulate the proliferation and regeneration of cells. In combination with exercise, your diet will help regulate blood sugar levels and correct insulin resistance caused by eating highly processed and high glycemic response foods that trigger a cycle of high and low blood sugar spikes.

We will learn the benefits of water and how much water you should take daily according to your body weight. Water is essential to every body system, including sleep quality, brain function, optimal performance, and mood. It hydrates the body, cleanses and detoxifies it, regulates body temperature, protects joints and organs, and transports oxygen and nutrients through circulation for optimal cell function. You may need to gradually increase your water intake until you reach the correct amount. I will take you through the steps you need to get there.

Every year after age 30, for most, you lose strength, stability, muscle, and bone mass. You can lose up to 5% per decade.[54] Exercise is the best medication to slow this loss. It benefits weight loss and reduces the risk of heart disease, diabetes, and some cancers. It boosts mood and can reduce stress, anxiety, and depression. Exercise improves your immune system by increasing the innate immune cells that fight infection. Any physical activity benefits your health, and I'll give you your next steps regardless of where you are today. Staying active reduces the risk of breast, colon, lung, esophagus, and stomach cancer. Get tips on the types of exercise you need and how much you should do every day to boost your metabolism, increase stability, and reduce the risk of falls as you age.

You will discover the benefits of relaxation and how to control stress and manage your state of mind with positivity and gratitude. We must have time for recovery, both body and mind. Keeping your adrenaline running at full speed is damaging to your health. Chronic stress can affect your digestive health and increase your risk of heart disease, cancer, autoimmune, diabetes, and mental illnesses such as anxiety disorders and depression. [55]

We need only a few things to stay alive, and eliminating waste is one of them. Not only must we eliminate through the bowels, kidneys, and skin, but we have toxins in our body that, if we can eliminate them, our health will surely benefit. The body eliminates toxins through urine, perspiration, and bowel movements. Daily bowel movements indicate the state of gut health, and gut health is vital to your overall health. You will learn how to monitor bowel movements and what to do to ensure a healthy gut, which is essential for longevity.

Longevity Secrets will be your guide to improving your health and longevity. You will get an easy-to-follow step-by-step plan for implementing these five pillars into your life regardless of where you're beginning. The fundamental question is, are you ready to take charge of your health? Deciding to change your daily healthy habits is the first step to experiencing the joy of a pain-free, healthy and long life. Let's get started.

2

SLEEP YOUR WAY TO HEALTH

Sleep is a non-negotiable pillar of a long, healthy life. Getting enough sleep is just as important, if not more so, as a healthy diet and regular exercise for optimal health. You are undermining all your efforts if you practice healthy eating and spend hours in the gym but don't get at least seven hours of quality natural sleep every night.[2] According to the National Sleep Foundation, adults require a minimum of seven hours of sleep every night for a healthy life.[3]

We are in a sleep deprivation epidemic. Most people get less than the recommended sleep, which is detrimental to their health and well-being. As a society that glorifies people who stay awake all night to work, study or watch movies with the analogy that you will sleep 'when you are dead' and equate sleep with laziness, it is easy to undermine the importance of sleep. It may seem obvious to most people that sleep is essential. But how many people heed the warning to burn a candle on both ends? Even without research, we know how we feel when we don't get enough sleep for a prolonged period. While getting enough sleep gives us an energy boost to be alert and more efficient. While most people treat sleep as a luxury, it is one of the critical pillars of longevity. According to the CDC, one in three adults does not get sufficient sleep.[3] Lack of adequate sleep affects productivity, can limit work output and has long-term health repercussions. Still, most importantly, inadequate sleep is the easiest thing to do for yourself; that's unhealthy. Sleep deprivation is detrimental to our economy and productivity and is linked to chronic conditions such as obesity, heart disease, depression, and type two diabetes, among others.[4]

Understanding the impact of sleep on your health will help you make healthier decisions. I will share information about the benefits of adequate sleep and how you can sleep your way to a healthier and longer life.

Why Do We Sleep?

Sleep is the most undervalued pillar of health and longevity today. We make it optional and view it as a luxury, yet the lack of it is harmful to the body. Inadequate sleep raises blood pressure, increases stress hormones, and affects the blood sugar balance. It also affects mood and increases the levels of inflammation in the body.[2]

Sleeping may seem trivial compared to the long list of work that needs to be done. However, the fact that we are asleep for a third of our lives shows how important sleep is for the quality of our lives. Adequate sleep is critical for the functioning of our physical and mental health. The brain and every cell in our body needs sleep to regenerate and enhance their function. Thus, they can be affected negatively by inadequate sleep, and this can have a detrimental effect on your health and productivity.[5]

I have worked with several patients who hadn't prioritized sleep. And I had been there myself before I decided to take charge of my health. I can confidently say that changing sleep habits and prioritizing quality natural sleep is a fundamental part of the work required to be a healthier version of yourself.

Causes of Sleep Deprivation

- Age: people above 65 years may have more trouble sleeping, unlike younger adults or children, because of changes to the circadian rhythm as they age or due to medical conditions.[2]

- Illness: Some illnesses can affect sleep, such as sleep apnea or restless leg syndrome that keeps you awake.[3]

- Poor sleep habits where you don't have a consistent sleep and wake cycle, like alternating shifts.

- Sleep cycles that are not consistent with your circadian rhythm, such as the night shift.

- Environmental disruptions, including blue or bright lights, nearby electrical devices, and noise.

- If your bed is uncomfortable or your room doesn't block light appropriately.

- Eating too close to bedtime.

- Drinking excessive alcohol.

Symptoms of Inadequate Sleep

In addition to the symptoms below, many others occur due to inadequate sleep. However, they may not be as noticeable to you, such as how your brain works. Sleep plays a crucial role in how you learn, for example. There's also evidence that sleep deprivation plays a role in Alzheimer's disease.[12] Some symptoms, which are illnesses, may be directly related to your sleep! [11]

- Poor memory [4]

- Irritability

- Lack of focus and concentration [6]

- Eye bags, puffy eyes, or dark circles under the eyes

- Impaired immunity

- Fatigue or sleepiness during the day

- Inability to focus [6]

- Low sex drive [5]

Benefits of Sleep

During sleep, the body rejuvenates. The natural body process performs an automatic cell renewal process to allow the detoxification of toxins and old cells and paves the way for the new class. The body is impressive, and it cleans up during sleep. When you sleep well, your brain is clear, and you can make better decisions.

In addition to giving your body the time and resources to recover, there are so many other benefits to sleep:

- You are more energetic and productive

- Improved concentration [1]

- Better memory and learning capacity [12]

- Fewer sugar cravings and able to make healthier food choices

- Improved immunity

- Cell renewal [4]

- Less risk of developing chronic illness [7]

- Longer life

- Lower risk of obesity [9]

- Lower stress levels [15]

What Happens When You Don't Get Enough Sleep?

More adults sleep less than seven hours due to increasing workload, technology advancement, and social activities. Many studies reveal the dangers of exposure to less sleep which increases your risk of illness. Several studies have shown how sleep is critical for immunity, memory, concentration, boosting metabolism, and other vital body functions.[12]

Lack of sleep has both long-term and short-term consequences. Short-term sleep deprivation can affect mood and productivity and increase the risk of road accidents and injury at work. On the other hand, chronic sleep deprivation leads to many health problems, such as obesity, asthma, arthritis, depression, stroke, heart disease, type two diabetes, and chronic kidney disease.[16] These chronic diseases have a role in premature death and the development and worsening of chronic diseases. It is clear that although it is easy to neglect sleep, it is also one of the easiest things we can do to improve our health.

Short-term Consequences of Inadequate Sleep

You are likely to have a lack of alertness and impaired mood. Sleeping less by even an hour can impact how you feel. A compromised mood can make you irritable and affect your relationships with other people.

- Fatigue during the day

- Impaired memory and inadequate sleep affect your ability to learn and retain new information [12]

- Low quality of life because you have no enthusiasm to participate in your daily activities [14]

- Drowsiness increases the likelihood of accidents while driving or at the workplace [15]

Sleep deprivation limits your ability to pay attention or make quick judgments to prevent accidents. It is the cause of many accidents and fatalities, and every time you drive when you don't have a good night of sleep, you risk your life and that of other users. Surprisingly drowsy driving due to lack of sleep has worse implications than drunk driving and causes more accidents.[12] Yet more people cut corners, sleep less, and are tempted to catch up with the latest TV show or signal one more work report instead of sleeping.

Long-term Effects of Inadequate Sleep

Fine Motor Skills

Numerous studies have shown that adequate sleep can enhance fine motor skills, reaction time, muscular power, endurance, and problem-solving skills.[17] All these skills tend to decline with age, which is one of the reasons why sleep is non-negotiable for longevity.

Sleep deprivation increases the production of cortisol, a stress hormone that causes anxiety and degrades memory.

Sleep is also vital in learning and motor skills development. Sleep increases neural activity related to learning new tasks. The brain picks up new skills during deep sleep and enhances memory formation. It leads to improvement in task performance and the ability to solve problems.[6]

Sleep contributes to successive learning because neural activation occurs during deep sleep. When learning new skills, the brain activates the neurons required to perform the skill. Consequently, the brain reinforces the critical cells needed for mastery when you go to sleep.[12] You then master the skill because the brain waves activate only the vital neurons required. Indeed, you cannot ignore sleep when you are trying to learn a new skill or healing after an injury and you're trying to regain movement control.

Sleep is fundamental for physical and cognitive ability and reduces the risk of injury. According to research that targeted elite athletes, sleep was a contributing factor to the athlete's mental health and performance.[6]

Cardiovascular Disease

Low sleep quality and duration increases your risk of developing heart disease.[7]

Heart disease is the number one killer globally and in the US. According to the CDC, 1 in 3 adults, 75 million Americans, have high blood pressure.[8] Sadly, the numbers keep growing, which could worsen due to more people getting insufficient sleep.

Did you know that the day after daylight savings ends, that is the day after we move the clocks forward an hour, and most people in the United States, Sweden, and about a third of the world get an hour less sleep? That is the year's day with the highest number of fatalities from heart attacks. Americans' increased risk for heart attacks on this day is 24% greater than on any other day simply because of the number of people getting an hour less sleep. Yet, the risk for heart attacks decreases by 21% the day following the fall time change when many get an hour extra sleep. [57]

Sleep is vital for healing and rebuilding the heart vessels and controlling some processes that maintain blood pressure. During sleep, the blood pressure goes down. Chronic sleep deprivation raises the risk of heart disease because your blood pressure stays high for a long time. People with stroke, hypertension, or coronary heart disease tend to impair sleep patterns.[7] Sleep apnea is an important marker for cardiovascular diseases like atherosclerosis.

Diabetes

A lack of natural sleep is associated with a greater risk of developing type two diabetes and insulin resistance.[10]

Sleep deprivation increases your risk of getting type two diabetes by 55%. WOW! Sleep duration of fewer than 6 hours every night affects the release of insulin and causes insulin resistance because it impacts how the metabolism works.[10] Furthermore, the quality and quantity of sleep affect the levels of hemoglobin A1C, an essential marker for blood sugar control.

The latest statistics reveal that more than 100 million adults in the US have either prediabetes or diabetes, equating to 30 million being diagnosed with diabetes. Most people with sleep disorders or an impaired wake-sleep cycle have a higher risk of diabetes.[10] The relationship between sleep and diabetes is dual-sided. While lack of sufficient sleep increases the risk of diabetes, having diabetes also worsens the quality of sleep.

Sleep disturbance also causes changes in the hormonal system and leads to fat accumulation in the body, which causes obesity.[9] Obesity is directly linked to diabetes. See how this vicious circle is directly related to a lack of sleep?

Insufficient sleep causes a slowdown of body functions such as digestion, heart rate, heart rate variability, blood pressure, and respiration rate. If you don't get adequate sleep, natural body maintenance does not occur, resulting in higher levels of unnecessary hormones, and increased basal metabolism, thus causing insulin resistance. Of course, this often results in diabetes. Once diabetes sets in, it affects your sleep quality.[10]

Consistent sleep loss causes metabolic changes such as increased cortisol and ghrelin hormones, reduced leptin hormone, and impaired glucose metabolism. As you might have guessed, these hormonal changes improve your chances of developing type two diabetes.[10] Ghrelin and Leptin are hormones that help with hunger and appetite. These changes also increase appetite, leading to obesity.

Are you connecting how getting the proper amount of natural sleep is directly related to the quality of your life? I assure you that it is also directly related to the quantity of your life.

Numerous studies reveal the correlation between sleep deprivation and a higher risk of diabetes. According to research, people who slept less than five hours every night had twice the risk of developing diabetes compared to those who slept seven hours each night. The study further reveals that too much sleep also predisposes you to diabetes since people who slept more than 8 hours a day were three times at risk compared to those who slept for seven hours.[10] I'm not suggesting getting too much sleep, but instead getting the right amount of sleep. Furthermore, people who work night shifts have a higher risk of developing diabetes than those who work day shifts.[9]

Optimizing your sleep is essential to improving your blood sugar levels if you have type two diabetes. Lack of sleep affects glucose metabolism. Just six nights of sleep loss causes decreased glucose tolerance, while sleeping less than five and a half hours for 14 days reduces insulin sensitivity, activates an inflammatory response, worsens inflammation, and you guessed it, contributes to the development of diabetes.[10]

Mental Health

Let's move on from diabetes and address your mental health. Mental health concerns are strongly linked to poor sleep quality and sleeping disorders. Have you ever noticed that you are more irritable when you don't sleep well at night? Well, interruptions in your sleep can affect your mood the next day. Chronic insomnia can predispose you to depression.

Studies show a correlation between sleep disturbances and anxiety and depression. People with anxiety or depression often have more significant trouble sleeping and are at higher risk of struggling with sleep disorders such as insomnia.[11] Poor sleep affects the ability to regulate emotions and may make you more vulnerable to anxiety and depression.[13] People overwhelmed with family or financial troubles often have difficulty sleeping or may wake up several times at night. Managing stress or seeking help if you have depression is the first step to correcting the issue, reducing sleep disturbance, and helping you improve the quality of sleep.

Insufficient sleep affects hormone production. Lack of adequate sleep increases the level of the stress hormone cortisol. High cortisol levels break down collagen vital for smooth skin, thus increasing your risk of wrinkles.[16]

Sleep and Your Brain

Cognition, memory, concentration, productivity, and performance are all negatively affected by sleep deprivation.[6] The list of detriments associated with a lack of adequate sleep goes on and on!

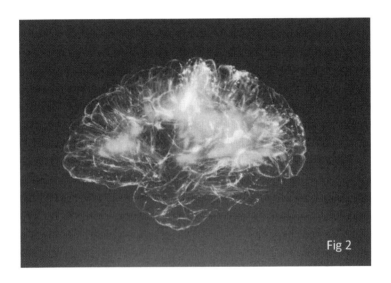

Fig 2

It is easier to retain new knowledge after a good night's sleep, just as it is challenging to learn without adequate sleep. According to research, sleep plays a vital role in memory and learning. The relationship between optimal sleep and memory is a complex phenomenon. The quality and quantity of sleep improves learning by consolidating memory and improving focus.[6] The brain consolidates the information while you sleep when you are introduced to new information. Thus, lack of sleep makes learning and retaining new information harder.

Sleep is essential to the brain, just as nutrition is to the body. Lack of adequate sleep affects the neurons' function, hinders regeneration, and impacts your performance because the brain is active all day when you are awake, and the neurons get tired. That's why you have trouble concentrating and remembering critical information. Natural sleep is an effortless and free pill to enhance optimal brain function.[12]

Glymphatic System

According to Harvard Health, sleep enhances the natural brain cleaning system, where the cerebrospinal fluid rushes through the brain and cleans beta-amyloid protein that causes damage to brain cells. The waste-elimination system is called the glymphatic system. It uses the cerebrospinal fluid to flush out the toxins accumulated in the brain and spinal cord. The brain can only do this when you are asleep.[16]

In addition to eliminating waste from the central nervous system, the glymphatic system is believed to help deliver glucose, amino acids, and lipids. The fascinating fact about this system is that it can only function during sleep and is dormant while you are awake.

Losing just one night of sleep can increase beta-amyloid levels to higher levels than usual, allowing the protein to accumulate in the brain. The worst part is that chronic sleep deprivation can interfere with brain function and make it vulnerable to developing Alzheimer's disease.[12]

Sleep improves memory recall after learning and can also reduce mental fatigue. When you sleep, the brain can recharge, eliminate toxins accumulated during the day, and perform optimal functions. Lack of sleep causes a build-up of toxins in the brain, which impacts your judgment and cognitive capability.[12]

Lack of sleep affects the brain just like if you were intoxicated with alcohol, which can impair your judgment and affect productivity at work.

Overweight and Obesity

Sleeping less than seven hours per night increases the risk of weight gain. Sleep affects metabolism and the hormones that control the feeling of hunger and satiety—chronic sleep deprivation results in metabolic changes that cause weight gain. People who sleep for a shorter duration have a higher risk of being overweight or obese.

Inadequate sleep can affect the release of insulin and cause increased storage of fat and thus leading to weight gain, a risk factor for type two diabetes. Here we go again with the diabetes connection.

Lack of sleep also causes the body to produce less leptin which helps to increase the feeling of fullness and produce more ghrelin hormone that stimulates hunger. Thus, making it harder to stick with healthier food choices and exercise routines.[9]

Numerous studies show that people who worked night shifts had three times higher risk of obesity than those who worked day shifts.[9] Working the night shift makes it very difficult to get adequate quality sleep because your sleep cycle conflicts with your natural circadian rhythm, which has a cortisol peak in the morning and melatonin peaking at night. The night shift workers had lower sleep duration, and inadequate sleep predisposed them to obesity. [56]

Social Relationships

Getting the proper amount of sleep may be vital in improving your relationships with others and helping you become more social.

Did you know that poor sleep can ruin your social life? Sleep loss affects the part of the brain that encourages standard social engagement. When you are sleep deprived, you tend to feel lonelier and more anxious in social settings. What's worse is that it alienates you from others because a well-rested person may notice your emotions and avoid you.[14] Thus, you become more alienated. This becomes a vicious cycle of loneliness. The less sleep you get, the less you want to interact with other people and the less they want to interact with you.

Sleep deprivation and the ability to control your emotions are related. When you have sleep disturbance, you tend to react more, affecting how you respond to others in the social setup. As we have seen above, lack of sleep also causes the rise of stress hormones. The relationship between depression and sleep is a vicious cycle. While sleep disturbance can be a symptom of depression, it can also be a cause.[13] Sufficient sleep is essential to prevent depression and negative emotions.

Inflammation

Poor sleep can also have a significant effect on inflammation in the body.[16] The results cannot reverse by sleeping in on Sunday after denying your body sleep over the week.

Inflammation is a silent killer that contributes to developing several life-threatening conditions such as type two diabetes, heart disease, stroke, Alzheimer's, and most autoimmune diseases. Inflammation is a natural body's response to injury or illness to improve the action of the immune system.[16] The immune system triggers the white blood cells to release inflammatory molecules, such as cytokines, that attack pathogens and protect the body's tissues. It is a temporary process that acts as a defense mechanism. However, factors like lack of sleep can trigger the reaction to last longer than necessary, increase inflammation in the body, and increase the inflammation markers that correlate with diseases.

When you sleep, your blood pressure drops, allowing the blood vessels to relax. Sleep deprivation prevents your blood pressure from relaxing as it should, which triggers inflammation in the blood vessels. Lack of adequate sleep also alters the body's response to stress. Research shows that sleep deprivation alters the mediators of inflammation in the body. Furthermore, losing half a night of sleep for people with hypertension increases blood pressure the next day and increases stress markers.[7]

Immune System Function

Adequate sleep has been shown to support healthy immune function. Sleep is fundamental to all body functions, and the immune system is no exception. Consistent sleep deprivation increases your risk of infections, particularly respiratory diseases, and affects how quickly you heal.[15]

Sleep disorders or disruption of the circadian rhythm can interfere with the healthy function of both the innate and adaptive immune systems. Sleeping less than seven hours hurts your immune system, makes it difficult to ward off infections and slows wound healing.

Getting adequate sleep strengthens the immune system and helps you fight infections. It supports the immune memory and the ability to recognize and respond to harmful antigens.[17] When you sleep, your body goes to rest, and muscle activity is reduced, thus freeing up the immune system's energy for the automated disease prevention process. Consequently, prioritizing sleep will protect you from illness and strengthen your body's response to infections.[17]

Disruption of the circadian rhythm can increase the risk of severe allergic reactions. Acute sleep disruption increases your risk of infections such as the common cold. When the immune system functions optimally, there is a balanced reaction to immune system triggers.[17]

Do you know why you tend to sleep when you are sick? It is the body's way of consolidating all the energy toward recovery. The immune response induces sleep to slow down other body functions freeing energy so the immune system can get all the power to fight infection.

Quality sleep also boosts the body's immune defense and plays a crucial role in improving antibody response to vaccines.[16] Not that I'm a proponent of vaccines, but if you are going to get them, then also get adequate sleep before and after vaccination to improve the efficacy of the vaccines.

Do You Have Poor Quality Sleep?

Tight work shifts, deadlines, sleeping in a noisy room, or using electronic gadgets in bed can affect the quality of your sleep. Other factors can be medical problems such as pain, sleep apnea, bipolar disease, or depression, affecting sleep quality.[9]

Here are a few ways that you can tell if your sleep quality is poor:

- It takes longer than 30 minutes to fall asleep

- When you wake up during the night more than once on most days, and it takes you more than 20 minutes to drift back to sleep.

- Having breathing difficulties during sleep

- Feeling tired in the morning even if you sleep the recommended hours.

Circadian Rhythm

Your circadian rhythm is an automatic body process to ensure that your body has adequate rest. The body's internal clock works alongside the day and night cycle and controls your sleep and wake cycle. Everything from the immune system, gut health, hormones, and sleep is influenced by a rhythm in the suprachiasmatic nucleus (SCN) in the hypothalamus part of the brain.[17] It regulates all the body functions by coordinating with all the other body clocks.

The difference with the other body functions controlled by the SCN is that sleep is influenced by light and darkness. The rhythm is controlled by a biological process that releases hormones that regulate sleep. In the evening, when the light begins to fade into darkness, the body produces more melatonin hormone to help you fall asleep and less melatonin in the morning when you are exposed to light to make you wake up.

The body's biological clock in the brain controls the 24-hour schedule of sleep and eating patterns. Ideally, the body is supposed to sleep when night falls and wakes when the sun rises. However, some factors can affect the rhythm and thus impact your sleep patterns. Exposure to light, exercise, temperature, and diseases such as depression, affect the biological clock.

When your sleep schedule is synched with your circadian rhythm, you get optimized sleep, increased productivity, and overall wellness. Although rhythm impacts appetite and eating patterns, we talk about sleep here. With an impaired rhythm, the body's internal clock will not send the right signals to help you sleep.[12] You may also wake up in the middle of the night and have trouble going back to sleep. That is why you must avoid exposure to light before bedtime for quality sleep, as this interference can affect your sleep quality.

Your circadian rhythm can also go out of sync due to internal malfunction like hormone imbalance, disease, or external factors like work shift hours, staying late to work, looking at your lighted electronic devices, or watching a movie too late at night.[9] Therefore, going against the natural rhythm that has existed since the beginning of life is harmful. Before the invention of artificial light, humans would sleep at sunset and wake up at sunrise. The creation of artificial light has made us think we can choose when to sleep.

People who work the night shift conflict with the body's natural clock. Some people feel alert at night and can only sleep past midnight, thus waking up late the next day, or others, when they sleep early, wake up in the middle of the night, especially in the late years. Travel can also cause disturbed sleep due to the disruption of the rhythm.

If you are not consistent with your wake and sleep time, drink caffeine or alcohol close to bedtime, or are exposed to bright light or blue light from your phone or computer before sleep, as well as others I mentioned prior, it can affect the natural body clock.

How to Sleep for Longevity

We saw the impact of sleep on mental and physical health, work performance, and overall quality of life. Persistent sleep deprivation can lead to short-term and long-term consequences such as depression and heart disease. For a better and longer life, approach sleep without looking for short-term quick fixes like sleeping drugs. The good news is that a few tweaks to your sleep routine will improve your sleep quality. It is not just about the quantity of sleep but also about the quality of sleep. Addressing sleep problems early enough to mitigate the consequences is essential. Here are helpful tips to improve the quality of your sleep.

Make Sleep a Priority

It is easy to prioritize getting work done over a good night's rest. Now that you understand how important sleep is, you should treat it as a doctor's prescription. Ensure that you schedule sleep just as an important meeting. You need to break down your tasks so you don't have to burn the midnight candle at both ends to meet the deadlines. Prioritizing sleep will improve overall health, lower stress levels, and improve productivity.

Establish Consistent Sleep and Wake Times

Consistent sleep and wake times regulate your circadian rhythm and help you sleep better and wake up well-rested. Irregular sleep patterns interfere with the sleep-wake cycle, impacting the production of melatonin that aids sleep and the cortisol that helps you wake. A fixed sleep time, even during the weekends, will reduce difficulties even during the weekdays. Once you establish a consistent sleep and wake time, you may not need an alarm clock.

Limit Alcohol Consumption

Avoid alcohol a few hours before bedtime because it impairs the hormones that regulate your sleep. It interferes with the production of melatonin, which controls the sleep and wake natural cycle.[18] Consequently, it increases the risk of sleep disorders such as sleep apnea, which disrupts sleep patterns.

Have a Bedtime Routine

Making slight changes to your routine can improve how you sleep. Do relaxing activities such as taking a warm bath, listening to calming music, or reading a book to train your mind to slowly wind down for sleep and make it easier to fall asleep faster. Doing the same activities before you sleep trains your body to know when it's time to sleep, and it will be easier to fall asleep.

Control Light Exposure

Exposure to light affects how you sleep because it regulates the body's internal clock. It interferes with your circadian rhythm. The body is wired to wake when exposed to natural light, stay awake during the day when there is natural light, and fall asleep at night when it is dark. According to the National Sleep Foundation, 51% of Americans are exposed to light in the morning. If you're exposed to light first thing in the morning, waking you earlier than expected, you must also go to sleep shortly after dark.[3]

During the day, exposure to natural light signals your body to produce less melatonin. In the morning, spend some time, ideally in natural sunlight, to signal the body to stop melatonin production. Exposure to the early morning sun signals the body clock that it is morning and to wake up, and it will improve your natural rhythm. It also enhances the quality and duration of your sleep at night and lowers the time it takes to fall asleep.

Although natural light is beneficial during the day, it is not at night. The body produces more significant amounts of melatonin when exposed to the dark. If you continue to be exposed to light, like during the daytime, you likely will not produce enough melatonin to fall asleep. Therefore, limiting light exposure at night allows the body to make the necessary melatonin.

Sleep in a dark room to signal the body to release more melatonin that helps you fall asleep. You can also use blackout curtains to eliminate light from the outside, creating a dark environment for optimal sleep. Darkness signals the body that it is time to sleep, so give it darkness before and during bedtime.

When sleeping outside your home, like in a hotel, light from the night lights can affect your sleep quality. When I'm in a hotel room or other temporary location for sleep, I put a rolled-up bath towel under the door to the room to block the light from the hall outside the room. I use rolled-up towels to cover up other lights in the room that are difficult to shut off, like the light on the microwave, clock, or television. I even bring a clip to close the window coverings to block any additional light from entering, such as from the parking lot. You will notice a significant improvement if you sleep in a dark room.

What if you are a parent who must check up on your kids at night? If you must keep lights on during the night, use red or soft yellow lights because they have fewer impacts on your circadian rhythm. Avoid white and blue lights. Try a small yellow or red night light. Give yourself just enough light, not any more than you need.

Electronics Exposure Before Sleep

Most people watch television and use their phone or computer way close to bedtime. Exposure to the blue light emitted by electronic devices could be the reason why you have difficulty sleeping. The light exposure, just like in the daytime, makes you awake.

The gadgets emit blue light that causes the same reaction in the brain as the sun, which signals the brain to stop or slow melatonin production. The same happens when you use your phone when you wake up in the middle of the night, making it harder to go back to sleep.

Light is a factor with electronic devices and the electric magnetic field they produce. For quality sleep, turn off all gadgets at least an hour before bed and keep them at least five feet away from your bed while you sleep.[56] Keep your phones and devices away from your bedroom because if you have them, you may be tempted to jump on social media or check your email before you sleep. If you must use them, set your phone to night mode to limit the intensity of the light as you work to restrict their usage before sleep. You can also use glasses or install apps that block the blue light if you must use your gadgets. Once you make these small changes, you will notice how fast you fall asleep and how long you stay asleep.

Make Your Bedroom a Haven

Noise, light, and temperature can affect the quality of sleep. Invest in a quality, comfortable mattress, pillows, and bedding that maintain your ideal temperature. Sleep in a quiet and dark room with the right temperature to improve sleep quality. Also, remove the television from your room and avoid watching negative content before sleeping. Consider using a white noise maker if you have outside noises that wake you at night. Make your bedroom a haven for sleep.

Use of Relaxation Techniques

Meditation, yoga, massage, and breathing exercises, especially at night, can help reduce stress affecting your sleep and help you fall asleep faster at night. I will review many ways to add relaxation to your lifestyle later, and the perfect time for these activities is about an hour before bedtime. Relaxing the body and mind is helpful for sleep indeed.

Gentle activities such as listening to soft music or visualization can reinforce the signals to the body that it is time to sleep and improves sleep quality. Using white noise machines or essential oils can also be helpful. If all else fails, read a book!

Exercise Helps You Sleep

Regular exercise improves your mental, heart, and overall health, energizes you during the day, reduces sleepiness, and makes you sleep better at night. Regular exercise also helps to regulate your circadian rhythm. It is one of the five pillars of longevity, and I will give you all the information for exercise to fill this void if needed, even if you lead a sedentary life and sit most of the day. Incorporating simple daily activities will improve your sleep quality, and you don't have to go to the gym to get these benefits.

Although exercise benefits your sleep, avoid exercising just before bed as it can make sleeping harder. Movement causes stimulation, and doing it right before bed can increase alertness and the time you take to fall asleep. Therefore, schedule your workouts, preferably in the morning or 3 hours before sleep time. It's time to stop making excuses and start an active lifestyle. Your longevity and sleep may depend on it.

Afternoon and Evening Caffeine

Caffeine causes overstimulation of the brain, which makes it hard to sleep and can cause you to wake up during the night. A cup of coffee boosts your focus and alertness during the day but can affect your sleep when taken in the afternoon or evening. Stop completely or limit about 6 hours before bedtime.

How Dinner Can Affect Sleep

Appetite, sleep, and the circadian rhythm controls metabolism. There is a relationship between consistent mealtimes, with the last meal being three hours or more before bedtime and healthier sleep. According to the National Sleep Foundation, people with consistent mealtimes have higher quality sleep and are 14% more likely to report lower stress levels that impact sleep.[4]

Avoid heavy meals, which can disrupt your sleep. If you eat a heavy meal before bed, you may experience restlessness, and you certainly will not give the body the quality sleep it deserves. Eat three hours or more before bedtime to give the body time for digestion.

Monitor Your Sleep Patterns

Keep a sleep diary, a journal, or a sleep app to record how much sleep you get every night and any cause of sleep disruption, e.g., stress at work. The sleep diary can help to analyze the root cause of sleep disturbance.

I would be remiss if I didn't mention that some disorders affect sleep patterns. If you have consistent sleep issues and these measures don't improve your sleep, reach out to a functional nutrition practitioner, functional medicine doctor, or endocrinologist, and they can test to determine if there is something more to your sleep challenges.

By making these changes, most people will notice an improvement in the quality of their sleep and the quality of their day. Each pillar also improves your others. An improvement in sleep makes it easier to eat healthily and to exercise, for example, and this gives you the motivation to make further improvements to your lifestyle.

3

EAT TO LIVE

The saying 'garbage in...garbage out' doesn't apply to what we put into our bodies. Garbage in means garbage in. Our bodies were never intended to have to clean up a continuous never-ending consumption of junk and toxins, and that garbage often remains in our bodies. It is costly for our bodies to function when we feed them unhealthy foods, and the results will show. What we eat and drink can affect our mental and physical well-being and lifespan. While genetics play a role, so does lifestyle, and diet is a crucial piece of the puzzle. Let's get into it.

I will be reviewing two specific food plans that research has shown increase years to your life: the Mediterranean Diet and what I call the modified Mediterranean Diet (MMD).

Candidly, the MMD is quite restrictive for most. Still, for those that want to do everything to live the longest and healthiest life possible, it is the diet I recommend and follow regularly.

For people who find the MMD too restrictive, the Mediterranean Diet remains the gold standard for living a longer, healthier life.

This chapter will explain both diets, what we should and should not include in our diet plan, how fasting plays a role in longevity, and other healthy nutrition habits. Let's get started.

Water – Another Non-negotiable

You might wonder why we address water intake now instead of jumping into the diet. That's because water in its purest form is non-negotiable for good health. It accounts for 60% (about two-thirds) of your body weight[19], and while you can go for weeks without food, dehydration can kill you in a matter of days or hours, depending on the weather and location. The quantity of water in the human body varies according to age, gender, muscle mass, and proportion of body fat.

Water is essential to every body system and for better sleep quality, brain function, optimal performance, and mood. It hydrates the body and cleanses and detoxifies it, regulates body temperature, protects joints and organs, and transports oxygen and nutrients through circulation for optimal cell function.[19]

How Much Water Should You Drink?

According to the National Academies of Medicine, women should consume about 11 cups (88 ounces), while men should drink 16 cups (128 ounces) daily.[19]

Because the systems in your body, such as your cardiovascular and lymphatic systems, have significant fluid requirements, the bigger you are, the more water you need. Just think about it, someone weighing 300 pounds has much more blood in their body than someone half the weight, and blood needs much water. Thus, I prefer not to generalize water consumption based on sex. It's more appropriate to relate water intake to body weight.

If you use the Imperial system, your water intake requirement is to drink one-half of your body weight (in pounds) in ounces daily. For example, if you weigh 180 pounds, you should drink 90 oz. of water daily. When using the metric system, you are to consume 10% above your body weight (in kilograms) in ounces of water every day. So, if you weigh 80 kilograms, you should drink 88 ounces of water daily.

It may sound unattainable to reach this fluid recommendation for some, but the good news is that the threshold includes fluids from many sources, not just water. Other liquids, such as soup, tea, coffee, and milk, contribute to your daily water consumption. However, be cautious when drinking fluids with caffeine because caffeine is a diuretic and can work against your water consumption, so keep your caffeinated drinks to a minimum. Moreover, you can get water from foods, mainly fruits and vegetables with high water content, such as cucumbers, celery, tomatoes, berries, and watermelon.[20]

I want to point out another thing about water consumption: there is such a thing as too much water. Too much water dilutes nutrients in your blood and stresses the kidneys. Indeed, drinking more than the kidneys have time to filter would not be good. The kidneys can filter .8 to 1 liter or 27-33 ounces an hour.[20] Unless you're perspiring away a lot of your fluid, you should not drink more than a liter of water per hour.

The kidneys cannot filter more water than a liter every hour, but that doesn't mean you should drink that much. If you drank a liter every hour you're awake, you'd consume about 4.75 gallons daily. That's too much for your body. As you drink more water, the blood volume increases, and the minerals and nutrients in the blood become diluted, causing levels to decrease. I suggest that water consumption be no more than double the minimum or the same amount of water in ounces as your weight in pounds.

Dehydration Epidemic

It is believed that over 75% of Americans are chronically dehydrated.[74] Normal body operations such as breathing, perspiring, digesting, and evacuation cause us to lose water. We must replace this water for the body to operate correctly.

Dehydration raises the accumulation of toxins in the body, which can cause various symptoms ranging from chronic weariness to premature aging. If you're thirsty, that's a sign you are already dehydrated. A properly hydrated body should excrete transparent, very light-yellow urine.

It is no surprise that our ancestors consumed more water than we do today. In the past, the only available fluid was water. Milk was introduced after the domestication of animals. As technological advancement came in, people devised beverages like alcohol, tea, and coffee for pleasure. Later, sugary drinks like sodas, sports, and energy drinks came in. The problem is that they are very high in calories, and the body struggles to regulate them.

With the many available beverages, it can be confusing to select the healthy option. Drinking plain water remains the best source of hydration. It is widely accessible and has zero calories. But what if you dislike the taste of water, as many do? Many people don't enjoy drinking plain water because we have been conditioned to expect a sweet taste in everything. You can enhance the flavor by infusing it with fruit or vegetables such as lemons, grapes, strawberries, oranges, or cucumber slices. You can also have herbal tea, but decaffeinated tea, preferably.

Some beverages may be harmful because they contain sugar, high fructose corn syrup, saccharin, aspartame, or sucralose. If you take advantage of our free eBook about sweeteners, as offered at the beginning of this book you'll learn why sugar and others are harmful. Beverages sweetened with sugar or high fructose corn syrup, such as soda, some juices, and fruit drinks, are high in calories and have little to no nutritional benefit. However, decaffeinated tea and coffee, low-fat milk or nut milk, or natural fruit juices are healthy without added sugar.

Benefits of Proper Hydration

- Colon Health: Water is essential for maintaining gut health and preventing constipation. Older adults are five times more prone than younger ones to have constipation.[19] Gut health is one of the five pillars of longevity, and water contributes significantly to our gut health.

- Water is also the key to keeping healthy, younger-looking skin if you want to keep it smooth, elastic, and radiant.[19]

- Water helps prevent inflammation and premature aging.[18]

- Water improves detoxification. The circulatory and lymphatic systems both have a significant amount of water. The more water they have, the more toxins they can carry to our liver and kidneys for cleansing our bodies.

Hydration Strategies

- First thing in the morning, drink some water. Our bodies are not just dehydrated after a long night's sleep, but they also contain increased concentrations of toxins. Before you reach for your morning cup of coffee, start with 8-16 ounces of water.

- Gradually increase your water intake if consuming less than the minimum recommended. For example, if your body needs 80 ounces and you have been drinking only 20 ounces, gradually increase your daily intake to 80 ounces. Consider setting the alarm to remind yourself to drink 4 ounces of water per hour, for example, and modify how much you drink each hour until you reach your required daily water goal.

- Avoid sugary drinks, alcohol, and caffeinated energy sports drinks. If you cannot, reduce them until you can and avoid them as you get closer to bedtime.

- Drink a glass of room-temperature water 30 minutes before your meals.

- Monitor your urine to notice the signs of dehydration and correct it early. You likely need more water when you see coloration darker than a very light yellow. If the color is crystal clear, you're drinking more than you need.

Water Safety

The type and quantity of water we drink affects our health. Rather than purchasing bottled water, which may include dangerous chemicals such as BPA (Bisphenol A), invest in a decent water purification system or choose BPA-free transparent bottles containing fresh filtered or spring water.

One of the most affordable drinking filtration systems I have come across is from Alta Water (https://atlawater.com/tamgall to get a discount), formerly known as Aqualiv. I have an Alta Water system installed in my home. You can install an under-the-counter system that filters out unwanted contaminants yet adds beneficial minerals back in, so you get mineral water at home.

Is distilled water healthy? Distillation is the process of boiling water, evaporating it, cooling, condensing, and converting the vapor (or steam) back into the water.[20] While distillation eliminates contaminants, it also removes naturally occurring minerals. Drinking distilled water dilutes the minerals in your blood without adding anything nutritional and may make your body excessively acidic. Prolonged usage could contribute to chronic acidity, resulting in significant health issues, poor energy levels, and fatigue.

Let's Talk About Fat

Let's talk a little bit about fat, shall we? Subcutaneous fat is the fat under your skin; visceral fat is the fat around your midsection and deeper under your abdominal muscles around your organs. Imagine fat between your intestines, stomach, kidneys, adrenal glands, and other organs at your midsection. Now imagine too much of it putting pressure on all these organs. Your small intestine might be thinking, 'what is this pressure I'm feeling? I can't do my job properly when I'm feeling squished.'

Your colon and other organs feel the same way and communicate with the brain. 'Hey, hypothalamus, can you help us out here? We need some more room to do our jobs.'

The hypothalamus in the brain, whom I refer to as the president of our endocrine system, tries to help and orders the pituitary gland to help the body deal with this stress. The pituitary gland sends an order to the adrenal glands, for example, for some cortisol to be released to help relieve inflammation in hopes it can help lessen some pressure. Now insulin must come and reduce the cortisol levels.

Can you see how excess visceral fat can cause hormonal havoc in the body? Visceral fat around your midsection tends to be more harmful than fat in any other part of the body because it is metabolically active and triggers the body to release hormones and inflammatory substances that are harmful to your health.[75]

Our metabolism declines as we age, resulting in fat accumulation around our belly, particularly for women after menopause. Living a sedentary lifestyle coupled with poor dietary habits makes it worse.

Here are some of the leading causes of excessive visceral fat:

- Genetics

- Simple carbohydrates

- Overeating

- Highly processed foods

- Too much unhealthy fat

- Alcohol consumption[61]

- Stress (excessive cortisol)

- Lack of sleep[61]

- Lack of exercise

- A leaky gut (hyperpermeability)[63]

A waist over 35 inches for women and 40 inches for men, representing excessive visceral fat, increases the risk for diseases such as diabetes, cancer, high blood pressure, heart disease, high cholesterol, high blood sugar, and stroke. Losing weight and lifestyle changes are the most effective ways to reduce belly fat. Eating a balanced diet rich in whole grains, fruits, vegetables, nuts, seeds, and legumes is essential. Also, controlling your food portions according to your body's needs is vital.

Metabolism and Weight

The term metabolism originated from the Greek word metabole, which means "changing," and describes all the chemical processes that occur continuously within our bodies to survive.[22] Nowadays, there is a lot of talk and concern about the relationship between metabolism and weight loss.

The good news is that you can determine your caloric needs using your basal metabolic rate (BMR) to help you manage the daily amount of food you consume based on your lifestyle.

You need a certain amount of energy in calories to keep you alive, so while you breathe, sleep, and maintain cardiovascular activities, the body consumes its caloric reserve, which is tied to everyone's basal metabolism.

Metabolic rate = the rate at which the organism expends its energy reserves. The Basal Metabolic Rate (BMR) is the energy, in the form of calories, necessary to keep the body's systems running at rest, such as heart rate, blood pressure, respiration, and body temperature.[21]

Consuming within your basal metabolic rate (BMR) is crucial for keeping a healthy amount of visceral fat and maintaining weight, especially after menopause.[21] Candidly, if you are overweight or have too much visceral belly fat, you need to consume even less than your current BMR.

The BMR comes in handy to determine the total number of calories you need according to your age, sex, weight, and height to lose or maintain weight or build muscle mass. The BMR varies with individuals since it is based on automatic body functions such as breathing and blood pumping.[22] However, a person with a higher muscle mass has a higher BMR because you need more energy to maintain muscles. Thus, you will burn more calories even at rest. If you want to keep your current weight, you should consume the same calories that you burn, while if you want to gain weight, you must consume extra calories than you burn.

You will combine the BMR with your daily activity to determine your total daily caloric requirement (TDCR), also known as Total Daily Energy Expenditure (TDEE). However, the figure may vary because your activity levels are not constant every day. There are online TDEE calculators that use the Harris-Benedict equation, which is considered to be the most accurate method to calculate. Some scales use bioimpedance that can estimate your BMR.

Here is how to calculate your TDEE manually:

Step 1: Determine the BMR[22]

- Men:

BMR = 66.5 + (13.75 x weight in kg) + (5.003 x height in cm) - (6.755 x age in years)

- Women:

BMR = 655.1 + (9.563 x weight in kg) + (1.850 x height in cm) - (4.676 x age in years)

Step 2: multiply the BMR with your activity levels to get the Total Energy Expenditure.

TDEE= BMR x Activity levels

Here are the five activity levels

1. Sedentary: You do little activity; you probably work from home or have a desk job.

2. Lightly active: 1.375 – You do light activities 1 to 3 days a week.

3. Moderately active: 1.55 – You exercise 3 to 5 days a week.

4. Very active: 1.725 – You exercise daily.

5. **Extremely active:** 1.9 – If you perform intense workouts or do heavy labors work every day.

The TDEE estimates the calories you should burn daily and helps to create a nutrition plan based on your caloric needs so that your energy expenditure is appropriate for your energy intake.[22]

To maintain your current weight, you should consume the calories according to your TDEE. To lose weight, you need to reduce your calorie intake by about 500, increase your activity levels, or do a combination of both. However, do not cut calories drastically unless you are under a doctor's supervision or working with a nutrition practitioner, as it will likely not work. Adaptive thermogenesis sometimes works against you. Start by reducing 250 calories between your food and exercise. Then, once your body adapts, you can reduce another 250 calories.

Under no circumstance should a woman or man consume less than 1100 or 1400 calories respectively without professional supervision.

To gain weight, you need to increase your caloric intake to build muscle. To get positive outcomes, consume an extra 250 calories comprising whole grains, healthy fats, and lean protein.

Ideally, the extra protein is consumed after a strength-building workout to support your muscles, and your extra carbohydrates are eaten before activities that elevate your heart rate to ensure you have the glucose available to support your cardio efforts. We'll review this in more detail when we discuss exercise for longevity.

Intermittent Fasting

Once you hit around 50 years of age, losing or maintaining a healthy weight is more problematic due to a slower metabolism caused by diminishing lean muscle mass.[23] Of course, the exact age at which you'll experience a slower metabolism may vary. However, everyone will have it happen to them one day. Once that day happens to you, weight loss or maintaining a healthy weight may no longer be about eating less and moving more; it may be about the timing of food intake…in comes time-restricted eating, commonly known as intermittent fasting.

In addition to being a tool to help you lose weight or maintain a healthy weight, intermittent fasting can help you live a healthier and longer life, as there are many therapeutic benefits of having times of fasting. Intermittent fasting (IF) has become more popular recently because of its health benefits like boosting the metabolism, preventing cancer, and improving autophagy and mental health.[23]

What exactly is intermittent fasting? It is an eating habit that alternates between the fasting and feeding phases. It is not food type restrictive as it doesn't prescribe which foods to eat but when to eat. Furthermore, it has different variations that you can choose from that suit your lifestyle. As a result, it is not regarded as a diet in the traditional sense but rather a pattern of food intake.

Here are the Three Types of Intermittent Fasting

- Daily Time Restricted Eating: A popular type of IF is the 16/8 rule. This gives you an 8-hour eating period and requires you to fast for 16 hours. For example, you can eat between 12 pm and 8 pm or 8 am and 4 pm. Most people prefer the 16/8 method since it is sustainable and easy to follow.[76] The other common approaches are 18/6, 14/10, and 12/12. The 18/6 means you eat within a six-hour window and fast for 18 hours. You can also do 12/12 as a place to start until you can implement the 16/8 rule. However, since most benefits of IF begin after 12 hours of fasting, I do not recommend the 12/12 approach for longevity.

- 24-hour fast: Here, you fast for 24 hours once or twice weekly. You fast from breakfast until breakfast the next day.[76] This method can cause extreme fatigue and irritability, and you should proceed cautiously or under a doctor's or nutrition practitioner's guidance.

- 5: 2 approach: In this case, you eat about 500 calories on two non-consecutive days of the week and eat regular healthy foods on the other five.[76] You can eat one meal each fast day or spread the calories throughout the day. When I work with patients in this approach, I prefer to give my patients the rule of consuming three calories per pound of body weight. For someone who weighs 300 pounds, you can get the same benefit with 900 calories, and it's easier for the individual. Similarly, if someone is 120 pounds, 500 calories are too many to benefit from this method.

Benefits of Intermittent Fasting

The fact is that fasting should not be viewed as just another fad diet. The process has far-reaching repercussions for our bodies that go beyond weight reduction (in fact, you can fast and yet gain weight if you overeat during your feeding period). Fasting has the added benefit of promoting health and lifespan due to the changes it creates in our cells.

In a nutshell, fasting cleanses our bodies and rejuvenates our cells, allowing us to live longer and healthier lives.[23] Of course, if you consume a nutritious diet, you may lose weight by fasting — but remember that you don't lose weight just by fasting, but by what you put on your plate.

Unless you're one of those few who, for medical reasons, cannot IF, I absolutely, definitely, beyond a shadow of a doubt, support the implementation of IF into your lifestyle for longevity and because of the outstanding health benefits it offers. Here's a little more detail on how and why IF works so well and the benefits you can experience.

Weight loss - Especially Belly Fat[23]

1. Fasting signals the body to use up the fat stored in the body, which is a good thing for weight loss. During your feeding time, ensure that you choose healthy foods and avoid highly processed junk foods if you want to lose weight. You can drink low-calorie drinks such as sugarless coffee or tea and water during the fast. Although I don't have any study that confirms this, I believe that Stevia can be used during the fasting period, and you'd still gain the full benefits of a fast.

2. Cell renewal: Scientists have already identified that severely cutting daily calorie intake or engaging in periods of food restriction stimulates the self-defense systems of cells. During fasting, the body performs a process called "autophagy," like self-cleaning, where the body expels the cells that are not functioning correctly or have been damaged. This results in cell rejuvenation.[23]

Fasting research has indicated that going longer without eating is preferable, so at a minimum, you can practice the 16/8 time-restricted eating approach. When we eat, the body stops caring about cell repair and instead spends much energy on digestive processes and food assimilation.[23] Therefore, fasting gives the body the time it needs to do the work it needs to do to improve its health.

3. Boosts Body Metabolism: Fasting has an additional advantage for persons over 40 or 50 years old, which is to combat the reduction in metabolism that occurs beyond that age (which makes many people start to gain weight). Our energy demands diminish as we age, and fasting not only boosts metabolism but it also can be a means to balance this account so that the individual can consume a bit fewer calories and maintain weight rather than starting to gain weight.

4. Blood Sugar Control and Improved Insulin Sensitivity: During menopause, several changes can affect a woman's metabolism, leading to insulin resistance and weight gain, especially at the midsection. This doesn't only occur with women during and after menopause as it is also directly related to obesity and genetics. Fasting boosts metabolism and reduces insulin resistance.

Consequently, lowering blood insulin levels and reducing fat storage in the body.[23]

5. Bone Health: Fasting improves hormonal function and bone health and reduces the risk of osteoporosis and pain from arthritis.[23]

6. Boosts Memory: Fasting is good for your mental health and contributes to improved memory, reduced anxiety, and better self-esteem.[23]

The list of benefits of IF is impressive. Here are additional benefits your body may realize once you implement IF into your lifestyle regularly:

- Decreases levels of leptin (your hunger hormone)[23]

- Benefits for those who have Parkinson's, autism, stroke, and mood and anxiety disorders [23]

- Increases levels of adiponectin (your fat-burning hormone) [64]

- Improves metabolic health [65]

- Diminishes depression [66]

- Decreases symptoms of epilepsy, Alzheimer's, and multiple sclerosis [67]

- Reduces inflammation [77]

- Lowers cardiovascular risk

- Improves brain function

- Increases longevity

- Reduces Blood Pressure

- Decreases incidence of diseases, including cancer [77]

How to Start Intermittent Fasting

If you wish to try the 16/8 approach, start slowly. Reduce the eating window while increasing the fasting time until you achieve 16 hours of fasting. Start by eating for 10 hours and fasting for 14 hours, for example, between 7 am and 5 pm, then break the fast at 7 am the next day. Or eat for 12 hours and fast for 12 hours. After the body adjusts, eat from 7 am to 3 pm and break the fast at 7 am the next day. This will allow your body to adapt to the fast.

For some, it is easier to skip dinner because the body requires less energy in the evening than in the morning. But if you are sedentary in the morning and your physical activity is often in the evening, then the noon to 8 pm time slot may better suit you. Ensure that your feeding/eating time makes sense for your energy expenditure, including your exercise hours.

You can use the 16/8 approach daily. For starters, fast for a few days every week or every other day until you adapt. Transition to daily IF when you feel your body is ready. You can only consume water, unsweetened coffee, and tea during a fast. Sparkling mineral water, like Pellegrino, is fine as well.

Most people experience increased hunger, irritability, and difficulty concentrating during fasting periods when they first begin to intermittent fast.[23] However, these symptoms usually go away once the body adjusts.

Is Intermittent Fasting Suitable for Everyone?

Despite the fantastic benefits of IF, it is not for everyone. Here are some exceptions. I highly recommend working with a professional if you are in any of these categories and wish to IF:

- People over the age of 65, particularly those with a chronic ailment

- People with hypoglycemia or diabetes should see their doctor beforehand.

- Underweight people

- Pregnant or breastfeeding mothers (IF is never an option)

- People with an eating disorder (binge eating, anorexia, or bulimia nervosa) should consult their doctor or be working with a qualified practitioner

- Children less than 18 years

A quick note on those with type two diabetes or hypertension, you can reduce or even eliminate your need for drugs. I have seen blood glucose and blood pressure return to healthy levels, so don't think you are stuck where you are. These are correctable issues for most, but I suggest you work with a doctor or nutritionist.

It's Time to Eat

Healthy eating habits boost your chances of living longer and enjoying each year with vitality. I'll explain what we should and should not include in our diet plan and how fasting plays a role in longevity and other healthy nutrition habits. Let's get started.

Although there are debates over what makes up an optimal diet, some factors, such as age, sex, and genetics, can influence health. However, nutrition is the most crucial factor you can control that influences whether you will be diagnosed with certain chronic diseases, and sedentary and frail in old age, or whether you will be active and robust. What you eat is one of the pillars of longevity that helps prevent disease and slow aging by empowering the body to rejuvenate, heal and protect itself. The type and quantity of food you eat can also determine your weight, sleep quality, and risk of chronic illnesses.

There has been an outcry over high-carb diets as the leading cause of obesity, and people are turning to high-protein and high-fat diets as a replacement for sugar. For those over 65, or those that are fragile, adding protein to help preserve muscle mass may be beneficial, however, for most, high protein diets are not sustainable and do not promote longevity.

What we need to do is to turn to complex carbohydrates and healthy fats instead. Plus, chronic caloric restriction is counterproductive. The contradicting information in a world that obsesses over body shape can be confusing. If you're over 50 years old, you have probably been told you should eat a low-fat diet. All this information is misleading and results in worse consequences. Reduced fat intake often results in increased refined sugar intake, which is detrimental to health. Your body has to get fuel from one or the other, fats or sugar; therefore, if you are on a low-fat diet, you will often get sugar cravings.

There are a few undisputable facts that improve longevity. They are applicable regardless of your food plan: adopting a nutritious lifestyle rather than a short-term approach is more effective, you should keep your body mass index (BMI) below 25, and it's essential to maintain healthy body fat and muscle mass applicable for your age and sex.

BMI is a calculation based on height and weight and indicates whether your weight is appropriate for your height. You can find BMI calculators online, and bioimpedance scales also estimate your BMI. You can also calculate yours by dividing your weight in pounds by your height in inches squared and then multiplying it by 703. For someone 140 pounds that 5'5", the equation looks like this:

$$140 / 65^2 \times 703 = 23.29$$

You can also calculate it by taking your body weight in kilograms and dividing it by your height in meters squared: Kg / m^2.

Healthy Fats

Fats are the body's primary source of stored energy in the human body, and they play a crucial role in hormone production and cell renewal. During the digestion of fats, the body breaks the triglycerides formed by fatty acids so they can be absorbed into the body. There are two types of fats:

Saturated fats... when the maximum number of hydrogen atoms is bound to each other. Animal meat and cheese have high amounts of saturated fats.

Unsaturated fats... fewer hydrogen atoms bound to each carbon. Includes monounsaturated and polyunsaturated. They naturally occur in plant-based oils such as olive, coconut, and avocado (not canola). Seafood also is high in unsaturated fat.

It's an indisputable fact that unsaturated fats are good for you, and saturated fats typically are not.

Protein

Proteins are the building blocks of tissues and muscles and are involved in critical cellular functions in the body. The body breaks down the protein you eat into amino acids absorbed in the small intestine and delivered to the cells to form new protein blocks. However, most people only need about 1/3 of our body weight in pounds in grams of protein each day, or .75 grams per kilogram of body weight, and a little more for those over 65 years of age, who have a challenge preserving muscle mass, or those trying to build additional muscle mass.

Because seafood and plant-based protein both are low or absent of saturated fat and offer unsaturated fats, it certainly makes sense that they would be recommended in any diet plan that's goal is longevity.

Carbohydrates

Carbohydrates are macronutrients essential in the body and are naturally found in most foods such as beans, grains, fruits, and vegetables. The primary role of carbohydrates is to be broken down into simple sugars that provide energy for the brain and body cells.[78] Without carbohydrates, the body converts fats into ketones as an alternative energy source. There are three types of carbohydrates:

Simple carbohydrates... also referred to as simple sugars. The unhealthiest simple carbohydrate is refined sugar. Even organic cane sugar is a simple carbohydrate. These substances are typically added to foods that don't give us many nutrients, like soda, desserts, and candy. Healthier simple sugars come from fruits, dairy, and vegetables.[78] These simple carbohydrates are a little more nutritious because they bring vitamins and minerals to the body. Examples include lactose found in milk and fructose found in fruits. However, all simple carbs are digested rather quickly and thus cause rapid changes in blood sugar levels and hence trigger an insulin response.

Starches... a form of complex carbohydrates. They have longer chains of glucose molecules which slow absorption. Starches include whole grains and vegetables like potatoes, corn, and peas.[78] Complex carbs take longer to be digested and absorbed since the long chains must be broken before they can be absorbed into the body.

Fiber... another form of complex carbohydrates. However, they are an indigestible part of some foods, including whole grains, fruits, vegetables, legumes, nuts, and seeds.[78] Fiber has many health benefits, one of which is that it is essential for gut health.

The popular belief that carbs are the only cause of weight gain and chronic illness has made low-carb diets more popular because they control blood sugar levels. Nevertheless, research shows that the quality of carbs can influence health. Some carbs are harmful to health; other carbs can improve health.

Another indisputable fact is that simple carbohydrates are usually not good for you, but complex carbs have many health benefits.

It's no surprise that when longevity is our goal, you must adopt a diet rich in plant-based protein, seafood, complex carbs, fiber, and unsaturated fats while reducing or eliminating the intake of simple carbohydrates and saturated fats. It is also not shocking to learn that I will be proposing just that.

The Mediterranean Diet

The Mediterranean Diet – labeled in 1960 by physiologist Ancel Keys and his wife Margaret in their book *How to Eat Well and Stay Well the Mediterranean Way*,[58] remains the gold standard for longevity. The U.S. News named it the number one healthiest diet in the world in 2022.[29]

The Mediterranean Diet has benefits for weight loss, reduces the risk of chronic diseases, and improves longevity. The diet includes a high intake of fruits and vegetables, whole grains, herbs, healthy fats from nuts, olive oil, and avocado, plus seafood a few times a week; moderate consumption of dairy products, eggs, and wine; and an infrequent intake of meat, processed foods, added sugar, refined grains, and trans fats. People who follow the diet have less risk of heart disease, type two diabetes, memory loss, and obesity.[29] The diet was initially followed by people who lived in countries near the Mediterranean Sea, such as France, Italy, and Greece, which is why it was named accordingly.

Benefits of the Mediterranean Diet include: [29]

- Weight control
- It's easy to follow
- Reduced risk of chronic illnesses such as heart disease, cancers, and type two diabetes
- Better blood sugar control is a non-negotiable for longevity
- Inflammation prevention
- lower rate of osteoporosis
- Slows down aging

Basic Guidelines of the Mediterranean Diet

Whole grains

Whole grains such as brown rice, quinoa, wheat, rye, buckwheat, oats, and corn are the primary energy source in the diet. This includes the use of these grains in whole-grain bread and pasta. Whole grains are rich in fiber and essential nutrients. The diet limits the consumption of refined grains or processed foods such as potato chips or crackers, white bread, white rice, white flour, cookies, cakes, processed meats such as sausage, fruit juice, soda, or any beverage with added sugar.

Fruits and vegetables

The diet promotes daily eating of fruits such as bananas, apples, oranges, and melon and vegetables such as broccoli, kale, tomatoes, cauliflower, and Brussels sprouts.[29] Consuming fruits and vegetables are associated with lower mortality risk from chronic illnesses such as heart disease.

Eat at least two servings of fruit and three vegetables daily. One cup of raw vegetables makes up one serving, while half a cup of cooked vegetables makes up a serving. An excellent strategy to meet the required veggies serving is to eat one cup at lunch and two at dinner or add veggies to your smoothies.

Protein

People who follow the Mediterranean diet eat more fish instead of red meat and have been found to live longer.[29] They eat meat only once or less per week; when they eat them, they only eat small portions. They replace meat with legumes such as beans, peas, and lentils. Poultry, eggs, yogurt, milk, or cheese is eaten only in moderation. [29]

The Mediterranean diet incorporates healthy seafood such as oysters, fish, shrimp, and clams. Seafood is rich in omega three and healthy protein that keeps you full and has a low glycemic index hence maintaining blood sugar levels.[29]

Healthy fats

Get healthy fats from fish, olive oil, nuts, seeds, avocado, olives, or avocado oil.

Nuts such as almonds, cashews, walnuts, and seeds such as flax seeds, sunflower, or pumpkin seeds are nutritional powerhouses. They provide healthy fat, protein, fiber, antioxidants, essential vitamins, and minerals such as magnesium and potassium.

The diet also allows moderate red wine, coffee, and tea consumption. People who follow the diet take a glass of wine with dinner.

As always, eat within your BMR or adjust it if you want to lose or gain weight, get the proper amount of water, and practice IF. In summary, the Mediterranean diet proposes:

1. Eat more fruits, vegetables, whole grains, nuts, seeds, legumes, fish, seafood, olive oil (extra virgin), avocado, and natural herbs and spices.
2. Eat eggs, chicken, turkey, cheese, milk, and yogurt in moderation.
3. Eat red meat, added sugars, processed foods such as sausage, and refined grains rarely, if ever.

The Modified Mediterranean Diet

There's no doubt that the Mediterranean Diet is a good start for longevity, but common sense can be applied to improving the diet, which I named the Modified Mediterranean Diet (MMD).

The MMD, which is the diet I regularly follow, considers these commonsense changes to the Mediterranean Diet:

- Elimination of processed foods, added sugar, refined grains, and trans fats. All these products are harmful to your health, as prior explained.
- Elimination of red meat and other high saturated fat foods, such as poultry's dark meat. Seafood and plant-based protein remain the primary sources of protein, with poultry white meat consumption occasionally.
- Egg whites can be eaten instead of eggs due to the difference in saturated fat.
- Milk and cheese products should be rarely eaten and ideally are low-fat and lactose-free.

The MMD is a healthy pescatarian diet most of the time, with some healthy dairy and poultry in moderation. It's as simple as that. By improving the gold standard Mediterranean diet by eliminating those unhealthy features it allows, the MMD is considered superior for longevity.

Continuous Energy Restriction Fast

Diets often fail because they require extreme changes to your diet and lifestyle. For example, if the MMD were to ask you to water fast for four to five days every month, that would be a crazy request. Fortunately, it certainly doesn't do that.

No one enjoys water fasting for prolonged periods. A water fast that long also has adverse effects as well. However, there are significant benefits to a prolonged fast that will aid longevity, such as improved regeneration and a reduction in autoimmunity, which is crucial to our ability to stay healthy. [82] Some additional benefits include living longer, improved cognitive function, reduced heart disease, and improved defenses against metabolic and oxidative stress.[83]

If you can get the benefits of a prolonged fast without fasting, would you consider it? Fortunately, there is a way. A continuous energy restriction fast (CERF) tricks the body into believing you're fasting so that you get the benefits of a fast without all the negatives because you will still be eating food. The body will continue to get the essential nutrients it needs to function optimally. This helps reduce or eliminate the adverse side effects of fasting. It has been shown to provide similar benefits as a Fasting Mimicking Diet®[84] which has significant research that indicates similar benefits of long-term fasting.[85]

Some people should not fast or should only do so under a doctor's supervision, so it is best to check with your doctor before long-term fasting or starting a CERF. If you're pregnant or breastfeeding, you should not fast long-term, even with a CERF. Additionally, if you struggle with maintaining appropriate muscle mass, are underweight, or have an eating disorder, now is not the time for a long-term fast. And finally, if you must expend significant calories during your day, for example, if you have a manual labor job or are training for a marathon, a prolonged fast isn't suitable for you either.

However, for most people, a CERF is healthy and low-risk. I complete a five to seven-day CERF quarterly because I'm convinced, based on the research, that it helps me manage my Crohn's disease and adds years to my life. You can consider longer if you like, but again, you should work with a qualified practitioner who can advise you on the maximum time appropriate for you.

I sometimes purchase a product from L-Nutra called ProLon, which technically is a fasting-mimicking diet, a form of CERF, or I create the meals on my own.

Prolon is a five-day fast. However, the first day is more of a transition day, which I tend not to follow. I reduce the contents of the first day to mirror the other days, giving myself five full days of fasting instead of four.

I follow a CERF more regularly by creating meals on my own. The rules I have developed through the years of working as a functional nutrition practitioner are as follows:

- You must determine your BMR as prior explained. Consume no more than half your BMR or 600 calories daily, whichever is greater.

- Consume no less than 25% of your BMR or 400 calories daily, whichever is greater.

- Follow a whole-food vegan diet without simple sugars such as fruits or added sugar.

- Eat low glycemic complex carbohydrates, such as tomatoes, broccoli, asparagus, cauliflower, beans, and other complex carbs.

- Eat healthy fats daily, including avocado, nuts, seeds, and olive oil.

- Supplement your nutrition with a multivitamin with minerals and an essential fatty acid.

- The day following this fast is a transition day; you should remain vegan that day but resume your typical daily caloric intake.

To experience the benefits of a long-term fast with a CERF, I suggest you bring these rules to your doctor, so they know exactly what you'll be eating before you start. I sincerely hope you take this next step and integrate a couple of times per year or once per quarter depending on your current health and goals.

I admit that the first two days of your first CERF are a little tough until your body gets used to it, and your first CERF will be more challenging than in future cycles. It gets easier each day and with each subsequent cycle, and it could easily make you significantly healthier and add years to your life.

4

EXERCISE TO STAY ACTIVE LONGER

Regular exercise is a necessary pillar of longevity and is one of the best things you can do for your health. Staying active makes you strong, reduces pain, and prevents chronic illnesses. But why is it so hard to keep a consistent workout routine?

We overcomplicate exercise by doing less because we approach an active lifestyle as something we only do on certain days and hang our tennis shoes afterward. We are supposed to be active throughout our day. It is not just meant to be a set time every day and remain sedentary the rest of the day. It is about keeping active throughout the day by finding more opportunities to move. Furthermore, most people think exercise is only necessary to lose weight even though what you eat plays a more critical role. Exercise has many more benefits than just weight loss. Staying active may not be easy, but if you make it part of your routine, you'll remain active longer, and it is worth it. The critical factor in making exercise work for you is to be consistent. Exercising hard five days a week and skipping the next two weeks doesn't work; instead, it increases your risk of injury. It is far more beneficial to exercise for at least 10 minutes every day for more benefit.

The CDC recommends 150 minutes of moderate activity and two days of strength training every week. Almost half of the population does not get this level of physical activity.[30]

Benefits of Regular Exercise

1.   Weight management

When combined with healthy eating, exercise tremendously impacts your weight. However, no amount of exercise can outwork an unhealthy diet, so you need to be conscious of what you are putting in your body. Exercise helps create a caloric deficit for those looking to lose weight, which means you burn more calories than you consume, thus allowing you to lose weight and maintain a healthy weight. [31]

2. Reduce the risk of heart disease, diabetes, and some cancers

Any amount of physical activity is beneficial to your health. Staying active reduces the risk of breast, colon, lung, esophagus, and stomach cancer. Exercise also improves cardiovascular function, lowers blood pressure, increases HDL (good cholesterol), and reduces the risk of heart attack and stroke.[31] Plus, it reduces menopausal symptoms such as hot flashes. [32]

Additionally, regular exercise improves your quality of life and fitness levels and controls blood pressure and sugar levels for those with a chronic condition or who are suffering from cancer. It also prevents nerve damage for people who have diabetes.

3. Boost metabolism

Aging brings many changes to the body. Post-menopausal women experience insomnia, body aches, pains, fatigue, weakened connective tissues supporting the pelvic floor, and a higher risk of osteoporosis. Most women exercise less, especially after menopause, which could worsen the metabolism decline that is common at that age.[32]

A low metabolism causes weight gain and difficulty in losing weight. Exercise helps to build muscle which burns more calories than fat, even at rest. Higher muscle mass and less body fat will result in you burning more calories, thus increasing your metabolism. [31]

4.   Improves mood and reduces anxiety and depression

You will notice a better mood immediately after a workout session because physical activity triggers the release of feel-good hormones. People who lead an active lifestyle have less risk of depression.[30]

5.   For strong bones and muscles

Exercise is essential for strong bones and muscles and especially for women after menopause, due to the likelihood of losing muscle mass. Physical activity keeps your muscles healthy and bones and joints in good condition. Strength training increases muscle mass, improves bone density, and lowers the risk of fractures.[32] Engaging in both strength training and cardio activities prevents the decline of bone density, thus reducing the risk of osteoporosis.

6.   Boost longevity

According to the CDC, regular physical activity can potentially reduce 110,000 deaths of American adults above the age of 40.[30] The best part is that increasing physical activity even by ten minutes daily is beneficial and reduces premature aging. Regular exercise increases your heart rate, making the heart stronger and prevents the risk of heart disease, which is the number one killer globally. [31]

Exercise also decreases transit time in your intestines, reducing the risk of colon cancer. Because activity also boosts moods, reduces depression, and helps you maintain a healthy weight loss, it increases your chances of living longer.[32]

7.   Improves energy and performance

Being active reduces the risk of injury and improves your ability to perform everyday functions. An active lifestyle after 50 reduces your risk of hip fracture and falls.[32]

8.   Cell regeneration

An hour of exercise is tough on the cells and makes them work harder. The result is that it forces the body to repair and prepare for the next strenuous activity.[30] No wonder you get sore muscles after a workout, but the more you exercise, the lesser the pain. The process of cell repair decreases age-related illnesses.

9. Boosts immune system

Exercise improves your immune system by increasing the innate immune cells that fight infection.[31]

Maximum Heart Rate and Heart Rate Zones

Before we get into what and how much exercise is recommended for longevity, let's review the different heart rate zones which will apply.

The heart rate is divided into five zones which act as the reference for the maximum heart rate according to the intensity level. The target heart rate per zone is determined using the maximum and the resting heart rates. [38]

Calculating your estimated maximum heart rate is pretty straightforward. Subtract your age from 220.[32] A 58-

year-old would have a maximum heart rate of 162 (220 minus 58).

Once you know your maximum heart rate, you can determine your target heart rate for each of the five exercise zones.

1. Zone 1 - Mildly Active/Recovery: 50-60% of your maximum heart rate [38] – warm up and cool down. This is where we spend most of our daily living while moving around but don't consider it exercise. Walking, laundry and household duties may be things you do daily in zone 1. You don't typically need to spend more time in this zone than you already are unless you are exercising for stability or have an extremely sedentary lifestyle.

2. Zone 2 - Low Cardio/Fat Burn: 60-70% of your maximum heart rate – fat burning and fitness training.[38] I like you to spend time in this zone while exercising for longevity, and it isn't likely that you will ever spend too much time here. I'll review in detail exercises for this zone soon. Here are some of the benefits of working in Zone 2:

a. Cardiovascular benefits include reducing your resting heart rate and increasing your maximum heart rate

b. Increases your aerobic capacity without building up lactic acid

c. Helps with weight management because the body usually burns fat instead of carbohydrates in this zone

d. Teaches the body to use fat more effectively as a fuel

e. Maintains glycogen (carbs) stores for high-intensity use.

f. Helps you to rest and recover more effectively

g. Increases endurance

3. Zone 3 - High Cardio: Endurance training and cardio are 70-80% of your maximum heart rate.[38] There are a few benefits of zone 3 workouts; the benefits don't relate to longevity. I'd prefer you take this effort back to zone 2.

4. Zone 4 – Low Anaerobic: Hardcore training is 80-90% of your maximum heart rate.[38] This zone utilizes more muscle which is one of the reasons I'm not too fond of this zone for longevity.

5. Zone 5 – High Anaerobic: 90-100% of your maximum heart rate – maximum effort.[38] I want you to spend a little time here for longevity, but I promise, it won't be much. Here are some benefits of working in zone 5:

   a. Allows you to reach a maximum speed

   b. You're strengthening your muscles and building up mitochondria in your fast twitch muscles, which is essential for eye-hand coordination as you age.

   c. It helps your body to learn how to process lactic acid.

   d. It increases your ability to take in and use oxygen proficiently.

The Building Blocks of Longevity Exercise

How should you exercise to improve longevity? Strenuous activity for extended periods puts much strain on the body and does not benefit longevity. Optimizing exercise for longevity is a precautionary measure to improve the quality of life later. It will determine whether you will be bedridden or can move around and remain active and have cognitive abilities like memory. It also gives you the strength and stability necessary to perform still the activities you enjoy, like playing with your grandkids, playing pickleball, walking without support, or engaging in other physical activities.

Even if you have not been active, it's not too late to start. You must start slowly with the usual daily activities you enjoy, such as walking. The good news is that increasing your activity by 30 minutes a week can tremendously positively change your health. Listen to your body and stop if you feel discomfort.

Longevity is related to mitochondrial function, which is enhanced by physical activity. Just like aging, a sedentary lifestyle makes us lose mitochondrial function. Exercise is the only magic pill that improves metabolic health and mitochondrial activity.[71]

There are four critical building blocks of exercise that we need to put into consideration to gain the full benefits of an active lifestyle: stability, strength, zone 2 cardio, and zone 5 anaerobic.[59] Any exercise for longevity must target these four key exercise components. Understanding these key aspects helps to optimize your workouts for a more full life as you age. Let's get into it.

Balance and Stability

Stability is the most essential building block of exercise and the cornerstone of your performance. Your heart rate will be in zone 1 or zone 2. In zone 2, the heart rate is 60-70% of your maximum heart rate. Using the example of a 58-year-old with a maximum heart rate of 162, her zone 2 heart rate target would be 97-113. Calculate your heart rate for zone 2 and work to keep your heart rate in zone two when working on stability exercises to kill two birds with one stone. Zone 1 is 50-60% of your maximum heart rate or 81-97 beats per minute for our 58-year-old.

If you're standing still on one foot, for example, working on balance, you'll likely be working in zone 1. And that's okay for balance exercise. But for Pilates and yoga, attempt to get to zone 2 for compound benefits.

As you age, your stability declines,[72] even if it is easy and automatic when you are younger. Simple tasks like sitting can be affected by stability as we age due to losing the pelvic floor's tension. Most exercises require both stability and strength.

Without stability, the body does not have the balance to stay upright when walking, cycling, or climbing stairs. It could also increase the risk of falls and injuries. Most people struggle in their later years with imbalance and have a higher risk of falls. A fall in childhood is a normal part of play, but in senior adulthood, it may cause broken bones that take longer to heal and affect mobility and deterioration of health.[31]

Some exercises can improve balance allowing you to move without assistance for longer. With the decline of muscle and bones that come with age, some exercises could enable you to perform activities like before since they support the alignment of your body.[34] According to Harvard

Health, some exercises can reduce falls by 37%, serious injuries by 43%, and bone fractures by 61%. [35]

Exercise programs seeking to improve balance also improve endurance and strength. The exercises make the muscles and bones stronger and more resistant to fractures. Furthermore, you can take quick actions with better balance because you are upright and have better coordination. Lastly, exercise improves brain function, making you think clearly and protecting yourself from falls.[31]

Yoga and Pilates are fabulous ways to improve your balance because they combine stability workouts with breathing, which helps to reduce stress and anxiety. Deep breathing also stimulates the vagus nerve, which has multiple benefits to your health, including gut health. Ideally, you include an hour of yoga or Pilates weekly. However, here are three exercises that will enhance stability that you can start doing at home immediately. If you're new to balance exercise, you may not want to do the exercises all at once. Also, use a chair or wall for stability if you struggle with balance. Do take a break if you are tired.

1. Single Leg Stance[35]

- Stand with your feet shoulder-width apart and arms at your sides as you face straight ahead. Maintain good posture and breathe normally.

- Lift your left foot a few inches from the floor as you shift your weight to your right leg. Bend the left knee slightly and remain in the position as you balance on the right leg for as long as possible. Start with 5 seconds and build up to 30 seconds. Hold on to a chair if you cannot do it without support.

- Put the foot down and repeat the same process with the right leg. That makes one repetition (rep).

- Repeat the same process three times. Keep doing the exercise daily until you can hold the leg for 60 seconds with your eyes closed for three reps.

2. Tree Pose[36]

- Do this yoga pose after the single-leg stance.

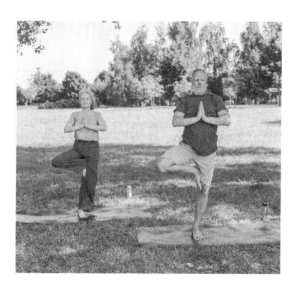

- Stand with your feet shoulder-width apart. Rest one hand on a chair if you need to and the other on the chest. If you can balance, place both hands together on your chest.

- Raise your left leg with a bent knee as you turn the foot inward. Place the sole of the left leg against the side of your right thigh and hold for at least 30 seconds. If you can't make it to 30 seconds immediately, hold this pose as long as you can and build up the time as your body develops more balance.

- Repeat the same on the right leg.

3.   Heal to Toe Walk[35]

- Find a location where you have a straight line you can walk and where you can put your hand against the wall if needed for stability. The wall is parallel to the line you're walking.

- Place your right foot on the line.

- Then, place your left foot in front of your right foot, so the heel is adjacent to the right foot's toes.

- Now, bring your right foot in front of your left foot so the heel is adjacent to the left foot's toes.

- Continue this for several feet, no less than ten steps, then turn around and complete the same thing in the opposite direction.

Strength and Muscle Mass

Strength training is another building block of longevity exercise. You'll be in and out of different heart rate zones reasonably quickly, so don't focus on your heart rate when strength training. Aging reduces muscle mass which causes a lack of strength and high mortality. A harmless fall in your 30s can be fatal in your 60s due to a lack of strength to support yourself. It is essential to preserve strength and muscle mass as we age because as you lose muscle mass, you lose strength. Additionally, strength training reduces your mortality risk threefold.[70]

Exercises that require lifting weight and grip things are beneficial to preserving muscle mass and strength. You can also use your body's resistance for weight-bearing exercises, such as squats, lunges, climbing stairs, pushups, deadlifts, and planks. The goal is not about setting records of how heavy you can lift but about the slow progress of increasing your strength.

Cardio workouts such as walking, running, or jogging are beneficial for health, but strength training is a significant factor in longevity and staying strong. According to research, 30 to 60 minutes of strength training every week increased life expectancy by 10-17%.[37] Wouldn't you like to add eight to fifteen years to your life? Ensure to do 30 minutes of strength training two times every week. Ideally, one session works the upper body and the other the lower body.

You also need to eat adequate protein to preserve muscle. In the previous chapter on diet and nutrition, we saw that eating low protein after 65 years can cause decreased muscle mass. So, support your muscles by eating protein 45 minutes to two hours after your strength-building exercise.

Strength training benefits include:[37]

1. Keeps the brain healthy and reduce the risk of Alzheimer's disease

2. Lowers blood pressure

3. Aids in weight management

4. Reduces the risk of heart disease: muscular strength reduces the chance of metabolic syndrome that causes excess abdominal fat and high blood sugar and blood pressure that cause heart disease

5. Improves insulin sensitivity and lower risk of type two diabetes

6. Betters chances of surviving cancer

7. Enhances mood and reduces stress and depression

8. Most importantly, it is necessary for mobility as you age

You need two 30-minute sessions per week on non-consecutive days. One day you'd focus on your upper body, and on the second strength training day, you should work on the lower body. The exercise type depends on age, gender, access to equipment, and current health status. If you're new to strength training, investing in a few training lessons might be best to get you started. Do your best to keep your heart rate in zone 1 or 2. If you get that heart rate into zone 3, don't keep it there long. Let it recover to zone 1 before continuing onto another rep or set.

Here are a couple of exercises for you to begin with for strength training without a weight room to get you started.

1. Lunges

Lunges not only help with strengthening leg muscles but also helps with balance. It's a strength exercise that helps improve your walking and running strength. [38]

- Stand straight with your hands on your hips.

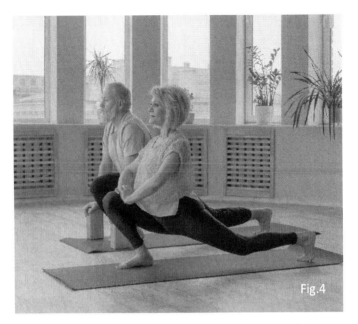

Fig.4

- Step forward with the left leg with a knee bent. Lower yourself to the floor until the thigh is parallel to the floor.

- Hold for 30 seconds as you breathe. Then return to the start position. Do it about 5 to 10 times for both legs as one set. As you get stronger, increase the number of sets. Make sure to recover your heart rate before beginning the next set.

2. Squats

- Your arms are to extend straight out in front of you

- Your legs are shoulder feet apart with your weight on the balls of your feet and heels, not your toes

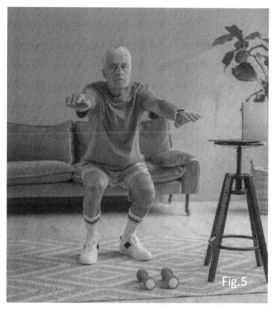

Fig.5

- Begin to bend your knees and lower your body as you flex your hips and push your butt back

- Your knees should be in alignment with your feet. They should not be extended further forward than your feet.

- Complete enough repetitions that your quads begin to burn. Then allow your heart rate and muscle burn to recover before beginning another set.

3. Forearm Planks:

I suggest you start with forearm planks, but if this is easy for you, you can do a standard plank that has you using your hands for support, not your forearms.

- Lay on the floor belly down with your hands under your shoulders and your forearms and hands on the floor

- Keeping your forearms and toes on the floor, slowly push your body up until your body is in a straight line from your knees to your toes.

- Hold this position for 30 seconds if you can and even longer as you get stronger. You may start shaking, and that's okay.

- Repeat this five times or as appropriate.

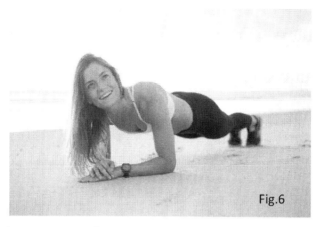

Fig.6

There is much more available regarding strength training if you have the equipment. But in the absence of equipment, use your body weight for resistance. Work your upper body one day, such as with planks, dead hangs, or deadlifts. And your lower body another day, with at least one recovery day. For example, your lower body can include lunges, squats, and stairs.

Zone 2 Cardio

Cardio training within zone 2 is another building block of longevity exercise. In zone 2, your heart rate is 60-70% of your maximum heart rate. The 58-year-old, with a maximum heart rate of 162, would need to get her heart rate to 97-113 to work out in zone 2 efficiently. What does your heart rate need to be? How do you plan on tracking it?

Zone 2 cardio, such as jogging, slow rowing, playing doubles recreational tennis, pickleball, low-impact aerobics, and brisk incline walking on the treadmill, make you more aerobically efficient. [39] To know if you are in zone two, you can measure your heart rate with a monitor. The heart rate should be high enough to make your workout efficient.

You need to do four 45-minute sessions weekly to increase your aerobic efficiency. [39] If you have more time, add an extra zone two session to enhance the benefits.

Zone 5 Anaerobic

You've likely heard of HIT or high-intensity interval training. This occurs during short bursts of high-intensity activity where your body can no longer use additional oxygen. Some refer to this zone as the Vo2 Max or the maximum volume of oxygen the body can use during exercise.[73]

If you run at a slow pace and use up 2 liters of oxygen per minute, speeding up means, you'll use up three or more liters.[69] If you continue to speed up and use 4 liters of oxygen per minute, you eventually plateau, where even if you work harder, you are not using more oxygen, and you've hit your VO2 maximum or the maximum volume of oxygen your body can use. This is where your body begins to use other forms of energy, and you can still go faster even if you are not using more oxygen. Repeating the recovery pattern at a low intensity after a short burst of the anaerobic or zone 5 is beneficial.[69] Most people spend little to no time in this zone. Yet a higher VO2 max or cardiorespiratory fitness max reduces the risk of death fivefold from chronic illnesses [59] which is why spending a little time here is required for longevity.

Admittedly, zone 5 training is the most difficult, but you don't have to spend much time here. Your heart rate must reach 90-100% of your maximum heart rate. Our 58-year-old would need her heart rate to be 146-162 in zone five.

Zone 5 workouts target the two energy systems, mitochondrial and glycolytic (which reduces efficiency as we age). Studies show that the level of VO2 highly correlates with longevity and a lower risk of diseases than any other variable.[39]

You only need one zone 5 training session a week. Ideally, your HIT is maintained for 4 minutes in zone 5 and then a 4-minute recovery. Work up to this if you can't do it now. Even one minute in zone 5 is better than none. Do this five times in a forty-minute session weekly.[39] Alternatively, you can combine zone 5 as you finish zone 2 by adding some high interval intensity of the last 8 minutes of the workout during each of your zone 2 training sessions. For example, in the final 8 minutes, you'll bring your heart rate to the max for 4 minutes and then recover the last 4 minutes. However, please don't start with high intensity (zone 5) because it will cause high lactate levels that limit lipolysis and interfere with the transport of fatty acids for the balance of your workout, which can cause cortisol anemia.[38] Combining zone 2 and zone 5, you must always do your zone 5 workout at the end.

For some, pushing yourself to the max for four minutes seems impossible. Don't think you have to do this on day one. In the concluding chapter, I'll give you some recommendations for all the pillars, including this one, that you can implement regardless of your current fitness level or health.

How do you get your heart rate to 90% of your maximum? The exercise includes high-impact workouts such as running, cycling, skipping rope, stair climbing, mountain climbing, or playing sports such as basketball or singles tennis. Work up to this workout as your other building blocks improve, and avoid these if you have injuries, low bone mass, or osteoporosis.

5

RELAXATION

And Your State of Mind

"The most important words you will ever hear are the words you say to yourself. So, make them positive. Make them kind."

~Marissa Peer

I came across this quote, which changed my view on many things and my perspective on how I think.

Indeed, this behavioral therapist and the author must have made an interesting observation of her personal life. Is it possible that she thought: 'My mind is a very negative place. I am always thinking about the worst and undesirable things.' But then, I'm sure she must have often experienced that deep sense of peace and happiness. And that's when she realized: '*What a difference it makes to say positive things to your mind!*'

Managing your thoughts play a crucial part in mental relaxation as well as physical relaxation. But managing your thoughts for relaxation isn't the only key to longevity. Controlling your thoughts, so they are positive and empowering, is also essential. If after completing this chapter, you find you are struggling with mental relaxation, meditation, mindfulness, and meditation, please consider my book *A Guide to Self-Mastery*. Details can be found in the Recommendations section of this book.

With the rising rate of depression and anxiety, it's more crucial than ever to advocate for mental health and daily routines that support physical, mental, and emotional well-being, especially after the COVID-19 epidemic. However, despite the pandemic, research shows that up to 73% of Americans indicate stress affects their mental health, while 33% feel highly stressed.[40] I can't imagine that the statistics globally are much different.

Imagine a difficult day when everything goes wrong. You have multiple deadlines, your child is unwell, and you have a board of directors' presentation tomorrow. In such conditions, your heart may beat faster, your breathing may become quick and shallow, and you may feel overwhelmed. These sensations originate from your body's 'fight-or-flight' response to a perceived threat. For some people, it happens occasionally. However, too much short-term stress might hamper your capacity to function correctly. In extreme circumstances, stress might cause death.[41]

The Difference Between Rest and Sleep

Work, family commitments, and stress keep you on your toes, and many never prioritize relaxation. We often only rest on vacations or holidays that last only a few days a year. It's crucial to get enough rest and quality sleep every day. Rest and sleep are vital for mental, emotional, and physical wellness.

Many people confuse rest with sleeping, but rest occurs while awake and has different outcomes for the body than sleeping. Resting the body is essential after intense workouts allowing your muscles to recover. Relaxing the mind is also crucial because allowing the hustle and bustle of the day to continue in your mind all your waking hours is hazardous to your health.

Rest might be mildly physical, like a stroll or yoga, or passive, like ten minutes of deep breathing or meditation. These regular habits can help you recuperate from physical and mental exertion. Prioritizing rest will also improve sleep quality, enhancing physical and psychological well-being.

Sleep, on the other hand, involves sensory isolation from our environment. Sleep affects cognitive function and immunological health and helps us refresh, recuperate, and refuel. It is also a critical factor in brain function, memory, focus, immunological health, and metabolism.[40] Unlike rest, your body requires sleep. You cannot live without it. Sleep-deprived people will fall asleep no matter what they're doing. We discussed in chapter two how to get quality sleep. Combining sleep strategies with relaxation will give you compounded health outcomes.

Benefits of Relaxation

Long-term stress can cause chest discomfort, headaches, digestive difficulties, anxiety, and depression, and increase your risk of heart disease, not to mention that it reduces your living pleasure. Here are the benefits of practicing daily relaxation:

- Reduced anxiety and stress [40]
- Improved mood keeping you happier
- Chronic pain relief
- Improved digestive health
- Reduced fatigue
- Less anger and frustration [40]
- Reduced blood pressure [41]
- Boosted immunity
- Lower heart rate
- Improved blood sugar control
- Boosted muscular blood flow
- More confidence in handling problems [41]
- A stronger heart [42]
- Reduction of stress hormones
- Improved focus and concentration [42]
- Improved sleep quality [43]
- Boosted confidence [43]

Relaxation Techniques

Relaxation is a necessary pillar of longevity that reduces mental and physical stress. It reduces long-term stress that increases your risk of heart disease. Learning relaxing strategies, whether your tension is out of control or under control, is beneficial and easy to understand.[41] For example, you can use them to relax before a performance, clear your thoughts to solve issues creatively, or compose yourself before a job interview. Regularly using these tactics could help you stay calm.

You should add several things to your calendar, such as meditation, yoga, strolling outside, listening to music, reading a book, or having a warm bath. Let's look at several relaxation techniques that help you calm down under stress, become more aware of your emotions, and redirect your attention. And the best part is that some are self-taught.

Deep breathing, gradual muscular relaxation, and centering can reduce muscle tension and moderate the fight-or-flight response.[41] This helps you think clearly and perform effectively under pressure. This section will explain multiple techniques and give you tips on how to get started.

Mental Relaxation:
Methods of Relaxing the Mind

How do you prioritize rest? Rest may not take precedence when you have numerous commitments. Sadly, you may lose out on relaxation's health advantages if you don't prioritize it. Find methods to relax regularly and put them into your schedule. Start de-stressing and boosting your health and well-being with easy relaxation exercises to improve mental health, focus memory, immune system, mood, and metabolism.[42] Your thoughts alone can manifest into physical illness. Your thoughts also determine your actions which can directly affect your health. Here are some mental relaxation techniques to control your mind and improve your long-term health.

Visualization

This relaxing method involves creating a mental image of something pleasant or positive to help you calm down. Use all your senses when possible during meditation for relaxation. For example, imagine yourself at your favorite resort on the beach, the warm sun on your body. Feel the warmth. Smell the ocean's salty fragrance and hear the crashing waves. Close your eyes and create a mental image and focus on your breathing. For an effective session, get to a quiet and peaceful place.

Meditation

Meditation is a mental relaxation technique that is effective for most people; committing to at least ten minutes daily will reduce anxiety and make you happier and more focused. It has long-lasting benefits to our lives and doesn't need any expensive membership plan or special gear. Although meditation is not the cure or everything, combining it with other relaxation techniques relieves stress and improves longevity.[42]

Just like physical fitness training, there are different styles of meditation. Try one for a couple of weeks and see the relaxation response. Meditation is an ancient practice dating back to 5000 to 3500 BCE in Indus Valley (now Pakistan and India). It is reported that archaeologists found images that depict people sitting in a meditation posture, now referred to as the lotus pose, sitting on the ground with crossed legs, eyes slightly closed, and hands resting on the knees. Also, some Indian scriptures dating back to around 3000 years ago describe meditation styles.[43]

Benefits of Meditation

- Improved blood circulation [42]

- Reduced stress and anxiety

- Lower blood pressure [43]

- You will feel calmer, grateful, and peaceful

- Improved focus [44]

- Better social relationships

You can use a meditation app such as Calm, or guided meditations on YouTube, in addition to my book *A Guide to Self- Mastery* to learn meditation. You only need to be in a quiet environment, and I'll get you started with the basics here.

How to Meditate

1. Sit calmly and quietly on a chair or the floor. You can even lie on your back on the floor or your bed, although I don't recommend lying on your back if you do so before bedtime or if you fall asleep easily.

2. Set a timer for about five to ten minutes if you are a beginner.

3. While sitting, close your legs or kneel as long as you are comfortable and can hold the position for the entire duration. While lying down, place your hands at your side, or you can put your hands on your stomach, heart, or one on each.

4. Pay attention to your breath as you inhale and exhale. Imagine it traveling to your lungs when you inhale and exiting your body as you exhale.

5. When starting, your mind will wander to other things. Pay attention to your breath to get back on track. Don't be obsessed with perfection. Instead, be patient with yourself and always come back to your breathing when your mind wanders.

6. Open your eyes and lift your gaze when the timer goes off. Pay attention to any sounds in your surroundings and notice how your body feels and any emotions you may have. Keep practicing until you can comfortably meditate for a minimum of ten minutes.

Types of Meditation

Some meditations can be done in alternative ways to what I've described above.

1. Moving/walking meditation

A moving meditation, also known as daily life practice meditation, focuses and calms the mind via rhythmic physical motions. This might be yoga, jogging, or as you do chores such as folding laundry, vacuuming, or yard work. This is an excellent approach to beginning a meditation practice by adding to the activities that you already do. [43]

2. Walking Meditation:

Walking meditation is, of course, a form of moving meditation. Walk naturally with your hands in a comfortable position. As you take the steps, count your steps up to ten as you pay attention as every leg lifts and then falls; start back at one again and pause once you reach ten. Focus your attention on the walking and return to it every time the mind wanders.

3. Concentration meditation

Like the name, this meditation style requires you to focus on one thing. It could be your breath, which is my favorite, repeating a single word or mantra, or counting the beads of a "mala," a string of beads counting up to 108. A mala has a larger bead that you hold on to as you move the other small ones between your fingers until you return to the larger bead again.[43] You can even repeat a prayer. If you notice your mind wandering, let go of random thoughts and refocus your awareness. You will get better with practice.

Another concentration meditation is a body scan, where you focus on your body. Start by feeling your feet on the ground with or without shoes. Start scanning your whole body in your mind, from the feet to the head. Focus on the different body parts and notice the sensations you feel.

4. Loving-kindness Meditation

Practicing compassion is a necessary skill for happy relationships. It makes both you and others happy. The meditations remind you that you deserve happiness, as do your family, friends, and everyone else. Start with extending compassion to yourself before you open it to other people. Once you have mastered compassion for yourself, show compassion to your friends, family, strangers, and enemies.

Meditate on the good things in your life and celebrate joyful memories. Recite phrases that reflect on what you wish for, such as "I am happy" or "I am peaceful," inhale warmth and compassion into your heart and exhale the same to yourself. Focus on one phrase at a time and bring yourself back when you get distracted. Lastly, close your eyes and visualize compassion reaching all the parts of your body.

Once you focus on yourself, wrap your friend or family member with loving kindness with the same mantra; 'may you be happy,' 'may you be at peace and free from stress or anxiety,' or 'may you be free from suffering.' This time, visualize the person's picture and send them warmth and compassion. Once you are done, do the same for a stranger you just met or someone not very close to you and wish them the same. Think of everyone who was kind to or inspired you, and repeat the phrases you did for yourself. Bring yourself back to meditation every time the mind wanders. Focus on practice and not perfection, and you'll master it in no time.

By now, you are so fired up with warmth and compassion, express the same for someone you dislike or are not on good terms with and wish them the same warmth with compassion.

5. **Breath counting meditation**

It is a basic meditation for beginners that monks initially did to increase their concentration.

To start,

- Sit or lie in a comfortable space. Gaze softly straight ahead and keep your eyes relaxed or closed. I prefer meditating while lying on my back first thing in the morning before I start my day. However, avoid lying if you fall asleep easily.

- Inhale slowly through your nose while gently pulling your abdomen out as if you were filling it with air. Pause for four seconds.

- Then exhale slowly through your nose while pulling in your belly as if to squeeze out the inhaled air.

- The idea is that you breathe in for about three seconds, pause for three seconds, exhale for four seconds, then repeat. Don't worry if your mind wanders. Return your focus to your breathing. Take a moment to let go of your thoughts, then redirect your attention to each inhale and exhale. Start with two or three minutes, then increase it gradually.

6.   **Box breathing meditation**

This meditation follows the same steps above. However, you will breathe in for a count to four, pause for a count of four, exhale for a count of four, pause for a count of four, and then repeat.

Continuous meditation practice helps you to learn to focus on your breathing and notice when your mind wanders. This technique increases attention and mindfulness because learning to pay attention to our breathing helps to focus on the present moment instead of memories or speculation of the future.

How Often Should You Meditate?

Daily meditation is the best way to manage your emotions and care for your mental health. Our thoughts control our lives. Thus, making meditation a habit will help to control unpleasant thoughts that cause anxiety, stress, or anger. According to research by Amishi Jha, a neuroscientist, meditating for 12 minutes five days a week improves your ability to pay attention.[42] Another study also reveals that practicing meditation for 13 minutes every day for eight weeks has long-term benefits such as improved memory, focus, and less stress.[44] Although this study was for eight weeks, my experience is that you'll begin to see benefits much sooner.

The duration should be realistic, practical to you, replicable, and enjoyable. However, you can start with five minutes and build up to no less than ten minutes daily once you get the hang of it. The body scan and deep breathing is perfect for those 50 years of age and above. However, try to test what works for you. You can combine it with physical relaxation, especially on your recovery days between your strength training days. We will go over some of the physical relaxations in the next section.

How to Make Meditation a Habit

Have you ever noticed how some actions come automatically? For instance, how you lock your door, move to the car and open the door and start driving. Do you ever think about how you will drive the vehicle? No, because it has become automatic since you have done it repeatedly.

Did you know that 95% of our habits work on autopilot? You don't have to think about them because repeated action reduces the sensory inputs into a default brain signal that works automatically.[42] Repetition is indeed the mother of skill. The brain converts actions that we regularly do from the conscious mind to the subconscious mind and makes the activities run on autopilot. That's why it is difficult to change behavior that you've done for so long.

First, make meditation a habit; you have to do it regularly. It helps to get executive control rather than running on autopilot, thus strengthening your willpower, mindfulness, and ability to make decisions. The more you practice, the more mindful you become. Start with three to five minutes every day to build the habits. Keep adding the time until you can complete a minimum of ten minutes, with the goal of more.

Perhaps you are wondering about the need to become mindful, yet most of our habits run on autopilot, or in other words, are performed unconsciously. The reason is that autopilot uses shortcuts and can make you do impulsive behavior that you're used to without thinking.[44] However, when you become mindful, you focus on the present moment. You don't dwell on the past or speculate the future; you can use rationale to know what is best for you instead of acting on impulse, which isn't always best. Shifting the balance to mindfulness practice will take some work, but through meditation, it will become easy.

Second, use reminders when you intend to practice meditation. For example, place the yoga mat in the middle of the floor, or somewhere you'll see it as you walk around.

Thirdly, constantly adjust what's working or not working. Maybe reminders, such as sticky notes, work in the short term, but the old habits return. You can try using phone apps for notifications or writing daily notes to remind yourself. Adjust what is necessary to develop this new healthy habit.

Lastly, use habit stacking. Combine what you do regularly with the new habit you want to adopt. For instance, practice deep breathing whenever you visit the restroom or when the phone rings.

Autogenic Relaxation

Autogenic relaxation is an internal method where you combine visualization and awareness of the body to reduce stress and relieve muscular tension[41]. You visualize something positive as you keep repeating words that help you relax, then take deep breaths to relax your breathing, reduce the heart rate or relax each leg or arm. I enjoy combining mental and physical relaxation with meditation combined with an autogenic relaxation technique relaxing my toes and focusing on feeling the pulse of blood running through my big toes, then my ankles, calves, knees, etc. I typically do this during meditation while laying on my back, eyes closed and no light, in silence.

Physical Relaxation

In addition to relaxing your mind, relaxing the body is also essential. Deep breathing, progressive muscle relaxation, and centering are three physical stress-relieving practices. These approaches help you handle anxieties before a presentation or performance and improve focus. Let's go over some of the physical relaxation techniques.

Deep Breathing

Deep breathing is a simple yet effective relaxation technique. It's a significant aspect of yoga, meditation, and the familiar '10 deep breaths' method to relax, and for a good reason. Combined with other relaxation techniques, such as progressive muscular relaxation and meditation visualization, it disrupts the body's fight-or-flight response and reduces stress and anxiety. [45]

Shallow breathing reduces your body's oxygen intake and might make you uneasy when stressed. Deep breathing, on the other hand, reduces stress, blood pressure, and heart rate. Deep breathing, or diaphragmatic breathing, is when you breathe such that your lower abdomen expands when you inhale and not just breathing with your ribs in shallow breathing. The diaphragm moves downward, pulling the lungs with it. As your lungs expand, it pressures your interior organs to make more room for them. Your diaphragm pulls forward as you exhale, helping your lungs expel carbon dioxide.[45]

Do a daily practice to master deep breathing. Sit in a comfortable place. Take a slow, deep inhale through your nose, and focus on filling your lower belly. Meditation is the perfect time to practice deep breathing.

Centering

Centering was adopted from Aikido, a Japanese martial arts practice. Aikido means 'unifying life energy.' It combines physical and mental ways to relax, channel nervous energy, enhance concentration, and remain solid and grounded during stress.[41]

Your spiritual center, physically, is found in your body in the umbilical nerve complex, known as the hara or tanden. In adults, the hara is about 3 inches below the navel. It's a mass of nerves associated with your intestinal mesentery, sometimes called your second brain.

This second brain is part of your autonomic nervous system, which is the part of the nervous system that controls involuntary responses like your heart beating, blood pressure, digestion, breathing, etc. It also impacts your fight-or-flight response. [41]

Centering relaxes the second brain, reducing stress and anxiety and improves mindfulness.[81]

You may center yourself in three steps:

- Become aware of your breathing and practice deep and slow diaphragmatic breathing.

- Focus on your center and take at least five deep breaths. Concentrating on your center helps you maintain balance and control while stressed.

- As you breathe out with each breath, release negative energy.

Centering takes practice to master, just like the other techniques. Picture your negative energy gathering in your center, move it up to your lungs, and allow it to leave your body as you exhale. Visualize pushing away all the negative energy, leaving you peaceful and silent. Try it as much as possible to be practiced before you need it.

Progressive Muscle Relaxation

Progressive muscular relaxation (PMR) involves tensing and releasing muscles from your toes to your head or vice versa in a quiet place without distraction. This approach focuses on progressively tensing and relaxing each muscle group to help you become more aware of the physical sensations. The technique consciously relaxes your muscles when experiencing fear or stress by interrupting the body's fight-or-flight response. [45]

How to do PMR

Tense each muscle for five seconds, then release for thirty seconds. Try to exhale as you release the tension or say 'relax' as you relax the muscles slowly.[45] Here are some ways you can tense your muscles. Do so for five seconds, release for thirty seconds, and then repeat.

- Keep your eyes closed tight

- As though yawning, open your mouth wide

- With your hands in front of you, firmly clench your fists

- Pull your shoulder muscles up toward your ears

- Bend your arms to tighten your biceps

- Pull your legs together as you sit and squeeze your thighs as you push inward to tighten the thigh muscles

- Contract your abs

- Curl your toes downward

After tensing your muscles, it's easier to relax them entirely. Without tension, muscles don't relax as well.

Improving These Techniques:
Physical and Mental

Physical and mental relaxation techniques work best together. As with centering, mental practices can enhance physical relaxation. You can use visualization combined with deep breathing in a serene environment to help reduce tension and lower stress. [45] You may combine physical practices with positive affirmations to transform your thinking and mood.

Here are some other relaxation techniques if you're looking for variety:

- Getting a body massage (I love this one)

- Tai chi

- Yoga

- Biofeedback

- Music/art therapy

- Aromatherapy

- Hydrotherapy

Lastly, regular exercise is another technique that reduces stress.[45] If you're following the exercise recommended earlier, you have likely already noticed how helpful it is for your mental well-being. If you haven't yet implemented exercise, fit in some simple workouts over a lunch break or after work. Include positive visualization or moving meditation with your workouts.

You can do some deep breathing at your desk or incorporate any of the activities mentioned into your day to boost your energy and reduce stress. Don't sit too long; stretch or take a stroll. Move about during your lunch break, stand when you're on the phone, or visit a colleague in person.

All these strategies work. Choose one to start and schedule a convenient time for it regularly. If you practice, the procedure will become routine. I have had success with all these techniques. Choose one to start or try a variety to determine which works best for you. The method will become part of your daily routine if you practice consistently. If you miss a day, that's okay. Start the following day again.

Learning relaxation techniques might help you notice muscular tightness and other stress symptoms. Once you recognize the stress reaction, you may practice a relaxation method when you feel it to prevent stress from getting out of control. Keep in mind that relaxation takes practice. It is a skill that takes time to learn and improves with repetition. Take it easy if you don't get it the first time and be patient until you master the technique. Don't allow relaxing to become stressful. We don't want to be counterproductive. Try another relaxing method if one doesn't work.

People with mental health conditions or unhealed trauma may feel emotionally uncomfortable during relaxation exercises. If you feel emotional distress during relaxing, discontinue. It may be a sign of something deeper that's going on.

Optimism and Longevity

A healthy, positive attitude can improve your health and add years to your life. Being angry, stressed, or depressed can easily undo all the benefits of the pillars of longevity. According to research by Harvard T. H. Chan School of public health, women with high optimism live longer than ninety despite their race or ethnic group.[46]

Although social factors such as race and ethnicity affect optimism, the benefits of optimism are the same across all diverse groups. Initially, the research focused on factors that increase the risk of sickness and premature death. Still, the findings implied that positive aspects like optimism were a better way to promote healthy aging and a longer lifespan across varied ethnic groups.[46]

A prior study found a relationship between optimism and living over 85 years old, considered longevity. However, the study sample was predominantly Caucasian populations. The results were the same when they included women from all races and ethnic backgrounds. This was a surprise because the other races have a higher mortality rate than the Caucasian race.[46]

The researchers evaluated data and survey answers from postmenopausal women in the U.S who were between 50–79 years old, and they were followed for up to 26 years. According to the findings, the most optimistic participants, who made up 25% of individuals, were predicted to live 5.4%

longer than the others. These most optimistic participants also were expected to live 10% longer than the 25% who were least optimistic.[46]

I'm convinced that a positive mental attitude is one of those non-negotiables for longevity due to the damage that anger, anxiety, stress, and depression do to our health.

The findings of this research mean that we should change how we view decisions that affect our health. Instead of focusing on the negative factors that affect health, we should also pay attention to positive aspects, such as optimism, which is beneficial to our health.[46]

Additionally, recognize that when you're angry or stressed, hormonal changes in your body do not benefit your health. Managing these emotions through the techniques I have shared contributes years to your life and significantly to your living pleasure.

6

GUT HEALTH

A Non-Negotiable for Longevity

The health of your gut is an essential pillar of health and longevity. Your gut not only is over 70% of your immune system, but it's responsible for ensuring that the cells in your body get the nutrients it needs and that the waste from what we eat is adequately eliminated.

The gut also plays a significant role in the body's detoxification. The kidneys and liver do the majority of the work. Still, the gut, if not healthy, can spill unnecessary toxins into the body, making their job more difficult and sometimes impossible.

Keeping toxins and undigested foods and fats from getting into the body starts with gut health, which is why having daily, healthy, formed bowel movements are non-negotiable for good health and longevity. Your stool is a leading indicator of the health of the gut and the effectiveness of the digestive system process from food ingestion, digestion, absorption, and elimination.[48]

In my life and my practice, I have seen and experienced how gut health is vital to good health and longevity. This section will detail the importance of maintaining a healthy gut and how you can go about it. Let's get started.

How Does the Body Eliminate Waste

The body eliminates wastes and toxins ingested through perspiration, urine, and stool to prevent them from causing health issues. [47] Optimizing your body's ability to eliminate waste through feces, urine, and sweat prevents the storage and re-distribution of waste products throughout your body, where they will likely contribute to further impairment of function and health.

Your GI tract is a selective barrier that absorbs what the body needs and is a wall to what the body doesn't need when functioning optimally. However, these functions can be impaired when out of balance, inhibiting proper digestion and elimination. [48]

Perspiration

Although perspiration doesn't have much to do with gut health, I want to touch upon it here because it's part of your waste elimination system. Perspiring regulates your body's temperature and is essential to remove toxins from the body. Allow yourself to sweat more through exercise or sauna therapy to promote longevity and well-being. Sauna therapy can be effective for people who don't perspire much to release toxins accumulated in fat cells.[47]

Perspiring also:[48]

- Improves circulation

- Boosts skin health

- Relieves stress and exhaustion

- Reduces joint pain and stiffness,

- Improves cardiovascular health

- Lowers blood pressure

- Strengthens the immune system

- Eases weight control

- Reduces cellulite

- Improves sleep quality

Urine

Adequate water intake helps eliminate toxins through perspiration and urine. Your urine should be light yellow, although the color can be affected by drugs or supplements such as Vitamin B complex. Your diet improves the kidney's ability to eliminate waste. Eating foods rich in minerals and plant-based makes the urine slightly alkaline, which optimizes pH and makes the wastes easy to eliminate. [47]

Bowel Movements

It's time to talk about poop. Irregular bowel movements signal a problem with the GI tract and are unhealthy. Regular bowel movements, versus constipation, reduce the time waste products stay in the body and limit the reabsorption of toxins back to the body through the walls of the large intestines. You should have one to three bowel movements per day that are easy to pass.

The Bristol Stool Chart gives the different types of poop. Ideally, your poop is formed like number four on the Bristol Stool Chart. Anything more solid suggests

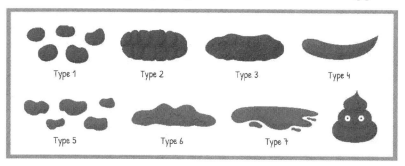

constipation or insufficient fluid in the stool, and anything looser signifies too much fluid. Both of which indicate that something is going on inside that isn't right.

Why are Daily Bowel Movements Important?

Bowel movements are an indicator of your gut health, which is significantly important to your overall health for a myriad of reasons.[48] Plus, bowel movements eliminate toxins from the body. Here are reasons why your daily bowel movements and the consistency of your poop are vital to longevity.

1. Your poop reveals if there are health issues

Your bowel movements reflect your health. They can indicate if something is going wrong.[48] Forget how people make fun of poo using poo GIFs and emojis. It's no surprise that doctors usually recommend a poop test to reveal what is happening when you have digestive issues. The poo always has the answer.

2. Regular bowel movements mean your organs are functioning optimally

The poop always leaves a clue. Your digestive health determines your overall health. Healthy poop often means that your diet is sufficient, your hormones are balanced, you are managing stress, your gut microbiome balance is good, and the digestive system is functioning optimally.[48]

On the other hand, unhealthy poop means you are stressed, have poor eating habits, don't drink sufficient water, have health issues or food intolerance, or are not physically active. You may experience low energy or a feeling of sluggishness, have a bad mood, or have trouble losing weight if you don't have regular bowel movements.

Monitoring Poop Quality

Monitoring your bowel movements is key to keeping your digestive health in check. Always check the color, smell, and appearance of your poop and record how often you have bowel movements. Compare to the Bristol Stool Chart and check how it looks most of the time.

The stool chart by the University of Bristol makes it easy to check the quality of your poop. We should opt for stool type 4 even though 3 and 5 are not bad. However, if you often have 1, 2, 6, or 7, you need to do something about it. The appearance may vary depending on what you eat, but it is good to notice how it appears on most days to get a sense of where it is in the poop chart.[48]

Here are some helpful questions.[48]

1. **How often do you have bowel movements in a week?** Having one to three bowel movements per day or as many meals as you have each day is ideal.

2. **Do you experience pain or have to exert effort?** It should be quick and painless; you need not strain and have to spend more time on the toilet.

3. **What is the color?** The healthy color is brown, although you may notice changes depending on what you eat. For instance, you may have green poo after eating leafy green vegetables or red after eating beets.

4. **How does it smell?** Although it can't be odorless, extremely foul-smelling poop can signal health issues. Also, check if it sinks or floats. Often it floats when you have a higher fat consumption or sinks when you eat more fiber. You should have poop that sinks.

The good news is that you can fix most issues if caught early.

What Your Poop Quality Says

1.   The efficiency of the gastrointestinal system

Poop appearance can reveal if the gut is working optimally or not. When you ingest food, digestion starts with your brain as you smell and think about food, then mechanical digestion begins by chewing. The muscular walls of the esophagus push food to the stomach through repetitive muscular contractions, also known as peristalsis.[48] The food is further broken down with the enzymes in the stomach and the early part of the small intestines. Nutrients get absorbed in the midsection of the small intestine, and waste products are pushed to the large intestine and expelled as feces.

The process is seamless when your gut is healthy and you have an appropriate transit time and healthy poop. When the poo is not healthy, it indicates that something has interfered with the normal function of the GI tract. Some factors that can cause gut dysfunction include hormone imbalance, spikes in blood sugar, malnutrition, microbial imbalance, and diseases such as colitis and Crohn's disease, which I'm intimately familiar with. Excessive use of antibiotics and painkillers disrupts the normal function of the gut. Your sleep patterns can affect the gut when your circadian rhythm is disrupted, such as through work shifts or jet lag changes.[48]

The problem with the gut is that it is rare to feel pain when dysfunction occurs. The problem is already blown out of proportion when you feel pain, such as when you have inflammatory bowel disease. So, just because you don't feel pain or discomfort doesn't mean all is well.

Research shows that the gut condition can affect communication with the brain and cause cognitive issues such as brain fog or changes in mood and an increased risk of anxiety. The gut and the brain constantly communicate through the millions of neurons that relay information. Therefore, gut dysfunction can affect mood, cause anxiety, and cause brain fog.[48]

You can also get physical issues such as an increased risk of uncontrollable weight gain, allergies, autoimmune conditions, joint inflammation, sleep disorders, kidney problems, and heart disease. Do you see why gut health is included as a pillar for longevity? Such conditions will worsen your quality of life and may cause premature death. [49]

2. Your gut microbiota balance

In the gut, we host a complex system of microorganisms such as bacteria, viruses, and fungi that benefit digestive health. They are present in the skin and mouth, but most reside in the colon. Unlike pathogens that cause illness, this system, also known as gut microbiota or microbiome, is actively involved in the digestion and absorption of food through digesting carbohydrates and the production of digestive enzymes.[50] We coexist with the microbiome that lives in our gut and feeds off our food but gives an array of benefits, such as the production of vitamins and serotonin hormone that regulates mood. Consider your intestinal bug colony as industrial workers who make you healthy.

We need the right balance for good health. Healthy poop indicates that the gut microbiome is balanced. In contrast, poop issues may indicate an imbalance of the gut microbiota that an unhealthy diet and lifestyle may cause, excessive use of antibiotics or alcohol, exposure to chemicals, digestion challenges, and stress affecting gut microbiota balance increasing allergies and food intolerance.[48]

The functions of the gut microbiome go beyond digestion. The gut microbiota is part of our body's defense system. The immune system not only protects us from airborne viruses and bacteria and prevents coughs and colds.

According to research, our microbiome's complexity may suggest we have more 'non-human' cells than human ones.[50] They boost the immune system and protect the body from pathogens by acting against harmful microorganisms. One study found that your gut has more immune reactions in one day than the rest of your body in a lifetime! This is because it has to counter-check everything we eat and react to foreign substances and allergens.

Our gut is a vital contact between the outside world and our bodies. The food we eat and its effect on our gut microbes are connected to the functioning of our immune system. By feeding the microbiota, we improve the immune system.[48]

However, a dysfunction in the balance causes a myriad of health issues, including metabolic, cardiovascular, and immune diseases, in addition to neurological disorders.[50] A healthy microbiome is also necessary for vitamin synthesis, digestion, detoxification, and a healthy immune system.

The good thing is that you can repair the gut balance and recondition the microbiome. The gut microbiome feeds on fiber found in vegetables such as broccoli, also known as prebiotic fiber. Fiber is not digested in the stomach or small intestine, so it gets to the large intestine, home to the microbiome, which ferments the fibers and causes the release of short-chain fatty acids, which have anti-inflammatory properties. Thus, reducing inflammation decreases the risk of heart disease, Alzheimer's, stroke, and others.[50]

3. **Is Your diet the problem?**

Your poop is waste from what you eat and reflects what is working or not in your diet. When you don't get sufficient fiber, you tend to get constipated, resulting in poo number one or two on the Bristol Stool Chart, which is hard to pass.[48] Apart from feeding the gut microbiome allowing fermentation to create the short-chain fatty acids which act as a fuel source, fiber also adds bulk to the feces. It makes it easy to expel the waste products after digestion, reducing the reabsorption of toxic wastes into the body.[50]

Diet and a balanced gut microbiota improve digestive function. During the fermentation of fiber, the production of short-chain fatty acids lowers the pH of the gut, making it the optimal environment for the growth of beneficial bacteria. Furthermore, fiber binds to fats and eases the excretion of hormones such as estrogen.[50]

4.   Are You Drinking Adequate Water?

We discussed earlier how getting the proper amount of water daily is non-negotiable for good health and longevity. The health of the gut is one of the reasons why. Remember, drink half your body weight in pounds in ounces of water daily.

Water helps to eliminate wastes in the body and keeps the gut environment optimal and functional. However, dehydration hinders normal function. Dehydration can worsen constipation even if you are taking enough fiber. Chronic dehydration can cause muscle cramps and dry mouth because the gut draws water from other areas to function.[47]

Consume more plain water and reduce the intake of coffee, sugary drinks, juices, and alcohol. We have covered water extensively in chapter three. You can always go back to the chapter and recalibrate your water intake.

5. Are You Managing Your Stress?

Have you ever noticed that you have trouble eating when you are stressed? This is due to the connection between the brain and the gut with the neurons that enhance communication. Too much stress or anxiety will alert the brain, digestion slows down, and there is limited blood flow and production of enzymes in the gut.[48]

Your poop will show you if you are anxious, fatigued, stressed, have sleep problems, trouble focusing, have headaches, depression, or are experiencing grief or sadness. Digestion slows down so the body can focus on dealing with the perceived threat making you anxious. Thus, you may get bloated, indigestion, and constipation.[50] It can work both ways, and you may get diarrhea when the stress is too much, as gut-brain communication can reduce transit time.

We have a chapter on relaxation, which helps significantly with stress management. Try relaxation techniques such as deep breathing, taking a stroll, yoga, or meditation, and make relaxation part of your daily schedule.

6. Are You Living a Sedentary Lifestyle?

Lack of adequate physical activity can affect your digestive health and the elimination process. Physical activity is crucial for keeping you in shape and improves your bowel movements. You can get constipated if you are not moving around.[47] However, you don't need to overdo it because it can stress your body and negatively affect bowel movements. Overworking your body reduces the blood flow to the gut, which can cause increased permeability, also known as leaky gut syndrome. Excess workouts can also cause sudden bouts of diarrhea during exercise.

As described in chapter four, have a balance of physical activity for good health and, as a result, improve bowel movements. Keep a journal to track if you experience changes on days that you work out. Monitor your stool output in the next seven days. Start with increasing just water intake and note any changes. Then make the other changes, like adding fiber one change at a time. The key to getting results is consistency. Always check your poo regularly and make the necessary adjustments.

I took a course through Functional Nutrition Alliance, and they suggested a *Food, Mood, Poop Journal*, which I implemented with patients in my practice.[51] The "Mood" is more about your body's mood, meaning did you feel bloated that day, have much energy, or were you fatigued? By using a *Food, Mood, Poop Journal*, you can begin to identify triggers causing challenges in your gut.[51]

Strategies to Enhance Detoxification and Elimination

1.   Limit intake of toxins

Would you knowingly ingest toxic material? Most would agree that they would not. I'm hopeful that after learning about these toxins, you will stop consuming them. The first step to detoxification is eliminating foods or products that can create havoc on your digestive health. Avoid trans fats and highly processed and preserved foods, as discussed in the *"Eat to Live"* chapter earlier. Eliminate eating or drinking from plastic containers containing BPA. Choose organic fruits and vegetables to reduce your intake of pesticides which your body must neutralize and detoxify. Also, consume free-range or grass-fed meat and poultry.[47] Avoid artificial coloring, flavoring, or sweeteners such as aspartame, saccharin, and sucralose.

Interestingly, you not only ingest harmful chemicals in diet alone, but many cosmetic products contain harmful chemicals that can disrupt body hormones. Minimize usage of such personal care products or choose those made with natural ingredients such as shea butter to reduce the chemical burden that the body must neutralize.[47] Although the body has a pretty good capacity to neutralize toxins, too much exposure makes the body use up more effort to neutralize instead of focusing on recovery and maintaining good health.

2.   Change your diet

Eat a diet rich in whole foods, fruits, and vegetables to provide sufficient fiber benefits to gut health and regular bowel movements and minimize processed foods. Both the Mediterranean Diet and MMD works exceptionally for gut health.

3. Drink adequate water

Water is beneficial in the elimination of waste products. Ensure that you stay hydrated.

4. Mindful eating

Eat slowly and chew food properly to make it easy for the gut to digest and control your food intake, as the gut will notify you when you get full. Focusing on your chewing and eating versus other things around you, actually improves digestion. Proper chewing aids in the effectiveness of the digestion process and nutrient absorption.[48] You should chew until the food in your mouth is the consistency of a smoothie before swallowing. Also, pay attention to hunger cues and only eat when hungry.

5. Improve gut microbiome balance

To fix an imbalance, you likely need to change your diet and include lots of fruits, vegetables, beans, legumes, and starchy foods such as sweet potatoes and cassava. These foods contain prebiotic fibers that feed the microbes so that they multiply and increase the defense in the body.[49] Ensure that the foods you eat are organic, free from pesticides that kill friendly bacteria, and limit processed foods.

To improve the gut microbiome diversity, eat fermented foods containing probiotics, which are friendly bacteria that give the benefits we have discussed above. Foods such as yogurt, kombucha, kefir, sauerkraut, kimchi, miso, tempeh, and plant-based fermented milk such as almond or coconut milk and pickles are good examples. Also, consider taking a probiotic supplement. [48]

Avoid the overuse of antibiotics that kill harmful and beneficial bacteria and affect the gut balance and the overuse of antibacterial soaps that eliminate even the beneficial bacteria from the body.[48] Planting a vegetable garden as exposure to soil bacteria can diversify your microbiome.

6. Monitor your poop

If you regularly notice any blood or red color in your stool and haven't eaten beets, go for a checkup. The presence of blood in the stool can signify health conditions such as hemorrhoids or, even worse, colon cancer.[48] Use the *Food, Mood, Poop* journal discussed earlier and recognize that type 4 on the Bristol Stool Chart is the goal.

7.   Manage stress

Stress affects the gut negatively, as seen in the previous chapter. Revisit the Relaxation chapter if stress and anxiety are an issue for you. Feel free to consider my book *Mental Health – Mental Peace* if the material I have for you here isn't doing the trick.

8.   Be active

Exercise not only strengthens the core muscles but also decreases transit time, which limits the amount of time the colon has to absorb water and helps prevent constipation.

Finally, if you need extra support— diet, stress management, or movement- you can always reach out to our clinic. One of my staff or I am always there to help.

9. **Improve Digestion**

As we age, we produce fewer digestive enzymes, and stomach acid regularly affects fat digestion and nutrient absorption. In addition to mindful eating, consider adding apple cider vinegar in a tablespoon diluted in eight ounces of water daily and digestive enzymes, which can significantly help when we're struggling with digestion.

Common Digestive Problems That Affect Longevity

Gut health doesn't always show up in bowel movements. So many people today struggle with digestion, which causes bowel toxicity and conditions that can affect digestive health, such as a leaky gut and inadequate stomach acid or digestive enzymes. Eating processed carbs and highly preserved foods are also significant causes of poor digestion, often resulting in a fungal or bacteria overgrowth, which can lead to hyperpermeability. This section will explore some of the challenges and their solutions.

Hypochlorhydria: Low stomach Acid

Hypochlorhydria is a condition where you have low stomach acid. It causes nutritional deficiencies such as protein, Vitamin B12, and iron due to poor absorption of nutrients. The acid is essential to activate stomach enzymes, enhance absorption of nutrients, help break down protein and boost immunity by preventing the growth of harmful bacteria and pathogens.[52] Since the acid is vital for proper digestion, its deficiency results in indigestion and poor absorption, leading to malnutrition and the overgrowth of harmful bacteria or fungus, which increase your risk of infections.[50]

Hypochlorhydria can induce persistent acid reflux, GERD, LPR, or heartburn. Insufficient stomach acid can cause gas bubbles to ascend into the esophagus and throat, transporting stomach acid. Even tiny levels of acid can be uncomfortable.[52]

Low stomach acid is directly related to improper digestion, especially concerning fats and gallbladder function. Now we have undigested food particles hanging out for too long in the gut. Undigested food produces short-term GI discomfort and long-term complications. Undigested food left to ferment in the GI system can cause small intestinal bacteria or fungal overgrowth (SIBO or SIFO). Low stomach acid makes you susceptible to H. pylori, which causes chronic gastritis and peptic ulcers.[52]

It's incredible how many of my overweight patients have low stomach acid. If you're unable to break down fats, your body tends to crave sugar, and here's the connection between obesity and hypochlorhydria.

Causes of Hypochlorhydria[52]

1. The use of medications to treat hyperchlorhydria or acid reflux symptoms such as heartburn or GERD causes even lower stomach acid and worsens digestive issues.

2. Bacterial infections that alter the stomach pH.

3. As we age, we produce less stomach acid.

4. Occasional stress should not be of concern, but chronic stress can lower stomach acid.

5. A diet high in sugar or processed foods can lower stomach acid.

Symptoms of Hypochlorhydria

- Since a leaky gut can be caused by hypochlorhydria, all of the symptoms of a leaky gut may also be signs of low stomach acid. These will be reviewed shortly.

- Nutritional deficiencies such as Vitamin B12, iron, and protein [52]

- Indigestion, GERD, or heartburn

- Bacterial infection [52]

Diagnosis of Hypochlorhydria

Hypochlorhydria is diagnosed using many tests. You can try a test at home and visit a nutrition practitioner if the home test is positive.

Taking an antacid will usually raise the stomach pH over 2.0, which is a given, meaning if you take antacids, you likely have hypochlorhydria. You can confirm the condition by using this simple baking soda test at home to determine if the stomach pH is too alkaline. Combining baking soda with stomach acid forms CO_2, which causes burping. To do the test, mix a quarter teaspoon of baking soda with half a glass of cold water and drink on an empty stomach. Set a timer to determine the time it takes you to burp. It should take, at most, three to five minutes. If it takes longer, or if it doesn't cause burping at all, you lack stomach acid.[52]

Correcting Hypochlorhydria

The good thing is that hypochlorhydria is reversible. Get a medical checkup before so the doctor can check for underlying issues such as infections, medications, or disorders of inflammatory diseases.

Here are some options for correcting hypochlorhydria:

1. Get a hydrochloric acid supplement such as betaine hydrochloride (HCL) that you will take with your meals. You will often use the HCL supplements with the enzyme pepsin to improve digestion. This supplement helps improve stomach acid levels and helps to return the levels to normal. This is the supplement we typically

use with our patients: <u>Pure Encapsulations Digestive Enzymes with HCL</u>

2. Treat nutrient deficiencies by taking a multivitamin. Low stomach acid levels can cause vitamin B12, iron, protein, calcium, and magnesium deficiencies.

3. Apple cider vinegar can increase stomach acid. Dilute a tablespoon in room temperature water and take it 30 minutes before meals. You can also get tablets if you don't tolerate the taste of apple cider vinegar.

4. Try these dietary recommendations to improve digestion while living with hypochlorhydria:

    - Eat protein at the beginning of your meal to stimulate acid production.

    - Wait 30 minutes after eating to drink water or fluids to allow the stomach to create sufficient acid and digest proteins.

    - Eat fermented foods such as yogurt, miso, and sauerkraut to enhance beneficial gut flora and control pathogenic microorganisms, which likely will be present with low stomach acid.

- Limit consumption of fatty and processed meals that are hard to digest with low stomach acid, have limited nutrients, and cause stomach inflammation, leading to reduced stomach acid.

- If you are a vegan or vegetarian, consider taking supplements for nutrients such as iron, calcium, vitamin B12, and protein, whose deficiencies can be more commonly caused by low stomach acid on a plant-based diet.[52]

- Eat small food portions and chew properly to give more time to activate the enzymes required to digest food. Chew until the food in your mouth has the consistency of a smoothie.

- Avoid eating late and eat your last meal two to three hours before sleep to allow time for digestion.

Improper Digestion

Improper digestion causes undigested food particles to putrefy, spoil, rot, and become toxic in your intestines. We just learned that hypochlorhydria could cause digestion issues, and I have found that other than a poor diet and stress, this is the leading cause of digestion challenges in otherwise healthy people. However, you should be aware of other causes of poor digestion.

Causes of poor digestion

1. Some gastrointestinal disorders, such as irritable bowel syndrome (IBS) and inflammatory bowel disease (IBD), can cause improper digestion, leading to symptoms such as constipation, heartburn, ingestion, gas, and bloating.[53]

   IBS affects about 10-15% of adults in the United States. IBD causes intestinal ulcers and has two forms; ulcerative colitis and Crohn's disease and affects over a million adults in the United States.[53] I'm one of those people (Crohn's).

2. Eating a diet rich in highly processed foods leads to increased stomach inflammation and lower stomach acid. They can also create a food source for candida in the small intestine, further impeding digestion. They often act as anti-nutrients. They take more from the body than they give.

3. Some medications, such as antibiotics and antacids, affect digestion. Opioid drugs such as morphine, codeine, and tramadol can also cause changes in digestive function.[53]

4. Dehydration can lead to digestive issues such as constipation. Inadequate water intake hardens stroll and reduces the number of bowel movements. Slowing transit time can increase the likelihood of bacterial and fungal overgrowths.

5. Chronic stress can also affect digestion and lead to inflammation and diarrhea. It can worsen the symptoms of irritable bowel syndrome.

6. People with diabetes also experience improper digestion because of elevated blood sugar levels.

7. I'm convinced that modified foods are challenging to break down. I have seen over and over in my practice; first-generation Americans have significantly more digestion challenges than those whose ancestors were American. And here in America, we preserve, modify, cross-pollinate, and deamidate food more than any nation I know.

Remedies of Poor Digestion

Lifestyle changes and home remedies can reduce the symptoms, but you should get a medical checkup if you have chronic digestive problems. Functional medicine and nutrition practitioners work with these types of issues regularly. Here are some helpful tips:

- Since we have seen the connection between stress and digestive issues, managing stress can reduce some symptoms. Get time to relax after your meals to relieve indigestion. Talk to someone about what is bothering you, and get enough sleep and exercise.

- Drink mint tea as a home remedy for nausea and indigestion: Peppermint oil can relieve symptoms of irritable bowel syndrome, such as stomach pain. Steep peppermint or spearmint leaves in a cup of hot water for about five minutes. Add some honey and a slice of lemon.

- Get the recommended exercise to improve digestive function: An active lifestyle increases blood circulation to the muscles, enhances gravity, and enables food to move through the digestive system more efficiently.[52] Go for a walk when you feel bloated to ease the feeling.

- Reduce gas from swallowing air when eating or drinking or produced after digestion: Trapped gas can cause stomach discomfort and bloat. Chewing gum, drinking carbonated drinks, or eating too quickly can cause increased gas. Limit your intake of foods such as apples, onions, broccoli, and yogurt that create more gas when moving in the digestive tract.[52] Gently rub your stomach after eating such foods to reduce bloating and discomfort.

- Eat fermented foods: Foods and drinks such as miso, kefir, sourdough bread, and kombucha contain beneficial microorganisms that benefit gut health.[49] We have seen how vital gut microbiota is to support a healthy digestive system.

- Eat more fiber: Fiber reduces cholesterol levels by binding to fats and preventing absorption, thus lowering the risk of heart disease. You should consume about 30 grams of fiber daily from whole grains, fruits, vegetables, legumes, nuts, and seeds. Ensure that you drink adequate water, which works with fiber to improve digestion.

- Keep note of your food intake and the symptoms you experience: Use a *Food, Mood, Poop Journal*.[51] Record your snacks, drinks, main meals, and the related symptoms. Once you discover foods that cause digestive issues, limit them from your diet and see if the symptoms improve.

- Limit trigger foods that cause issues with digestion: Limit foods such as fried foods, spices, highly processed foods, gluten, alcohol, caffeine, and acidic foods such as citrus fruits. Most fried foods are high in sugar, salt, and fats, making them hard to digest and causing gas and constipation.[52] Fried foods often use rancid oil or oil that has been heated so much that the oil decomposes, and this oil is challenging to digest and very harmful to our health.

- Take digestive enzymes: Because we produce fewer digestive enzymes when we age, it may be beneficial to supplement the enzymes to help break down food in the stomach, giving your enzymes more surface area to further break them down in the small intestine.

Leaky Gut

During digestion, nutrients are absorbed through the lining of the small intestinal wall into the bloodstream. A healthy person's gut has tight junctions with selective permeability to control what the body absorbs. As a result, they have good microbiota balance and have less risk of getting autoimmune and other diseases.[50]

On the other hand, an unhealthy gut lining develops wider junctions that allow pathogens, toxins, and partially digested food to penetrate through the lining and into the bloodstream and lymphatic system. This creates havoc in those systems and the immune system. The blood works to expel the unwanted toxins into the interstitial fluid, making the liver and the lymphatic system work overtime to eliminate the toxins. When the immune system works overtime, it proliferates immune cells to help, thus creating more immune cells and increasing the risk of autoimmune disorders. Studies demonstrate that changes in gut microbiota and inflammation can contribute to the development of chronic illnesses, especially autoimmune diseases depending on genetic susceptibility.[50]

The primary cause of hyperpermeability is digestion not working correctly. Here are some of the main culprits:

- Inadequate chewing

- Hypochlorhydria

- Gallbladder disfunction

- Reduced digestive enzymes

- Poor diet of highly preserved, modified, and processed foods.

Hyperpermeability is also called leaky gut syndrome, which increases the risk of illnesses such as autoimmune,

Alzheimer's, cancer, diabetes, food allergies, migraines, asthma, autism, lupus, and rheumatoid arthritis.[50] A leaky gut allows toxins into the blood, impairs health, and is a precursor to autoimmune disease.[49]

The relationship between leaky gut and microbiota balance

The microbiome in the gut affects several biological systems, including immunity. Gut microbiota dysbiosis causes autoimmune and bowel illnesses. It can cause an increased risk of arthritis and influence the onset and risk of developing lupus apart from a genetic predisposition.

People with a leaky gut have imbalanced gut microbiota with lower diversity. The right balance enhances the gut functions such as digestion, detoxification, synthesis of vitamins, and immunity.[49] This maintains a symbiotic relationship between the gut microbiome and the human. The gut microbiota forms a barrier on the gut lining to inhibit the invasion of disease-causing microorganisms.

Dysbiosis or imbalance of the gut microbiome can affect the integrity of the intestinal barrier, and it can become permeable, lead to inflammation, and provoke immune reactions. And if it stays in this condition, chronic inflammatory response causes the development of autoimmune disorders.[50] Although genetics plays a role in autoimmune disease development, the one sure way to prevent autoimmune is to take care of the gut, so this condition can't exist.

After developing an autoimmune disease, the gut must be tended to because it is evidence of dysbiosis. Keeping the gut in this unhealthy state leads to poor immune tolerance, which can worsen the severity of the disease.[50]

Leaky brain?

Because of the connection between the brain and the gut, some researchers believe that a leaky gut can cause a leaky brain, meaning a weakened blood-brain barrier. The blood-brain barrier allows the brain to get only the nutrients, water, and chemicals it needs and prevents the entry of toxins into the brain. It's another selective barrier we have. Excess toxins in the blood due to a leaky gut can get to the brain due to the compromised blood-brain barrier. When this barrier is compromised, it can cause neurological disease. Admittedly, there needs to be more research on these claims, even though we cannot refute them.

Symptoms of a leaky gut

Leaky gut symptoms include constipation, food sensitivities, chronic diarrhea, irritable bowel syndrome, gas or bloating, migraines, chronic fatigue, nutritional deficiencies, confusion, concentration problems, joint pain, skin issues such as acne, rashes, eczema, low immunity, sugar and carb cravings, arthritis, anxiety and depression, celiac disease, lupus, and Crohn's disease.[49] Wow! Can you see why gut health is a pillar of longevity?

Remedies to a leaky gut

The suggestions for maintaining a healthy gut and improving digestion include eating as recommended in chapter three. Still, a toxic bowel, resulting in a leaky gut, will likely need additional support. What you need to do depends on your underlying condition, such as limited beneficial bacteria, candida overgrowth, or food sensitivity.

In my practice, we help patients address the root cause of the symptoms of a leaky gut, discover their underlying difficulties, and establish a plan to fix them and prevent a recurrence. Often a total gut reconditioning is in order. Diet and lifestyle are typically the culprits.

Here are some helpful solutions:

1.   **Fix the gut microbiome.** One of the best ways to repair a leaky gut is to correct the gut microbiome balance and increase the diversity of beneficial bacteria, which will help to lower inflammation.[50] I have covered that in the previous section above.

2.   **Dietary and lifestyle interventions.** Eating more prebiotics, such as whole grains, fruits, legumes, and vegetables, avoiding highly processed foods and trans-fat, and making lifestyle changes such as increasing physical activity, stress management, and healthy eating can help.

3.   **Probiotics.** Eating probiotic foods and taking a probiotic supplement can also help restore the gut microbiota balance. This can be therapeutic for autoimmune diseases.[50]

4.   **Taking care of the villus:** We have little finger-like protrusions in our small intestine to increase the surface area for absorption called villi. I'm not going to go into extreme detail here, but if you have villous atrophy, you'll likely need to supplement these interventions with L-Glutamine and

others. This is where working with a qualified practitioner may be required.

Tips for Maintaining a Healthy Gut

Once the gut is healed and sealed, maintain a healthy gut by continuing to mind your gut.

1. **Diet:** Eat a healthy diet, such as the MMD or Mediterranean Diet, that helps to manage irritable bowel syndrome. These diets encourage a high intake of whole grains, vegetables, and healthy fats, aiding digestive health. Also, eliminate trans fats and processed, preserved, and refined foods. Eat organic as often as possible and avoid GMO foods.

2. **Healthy tea:** These can help to heal the gut naturally. Ginger is a natural herb that can help reduce nausea and inflammation and prevent ulcers and tumors. If you experience digestive issues, add ginger to your daily routine. Add fresh ginger to your smoothies or brew ginger with lemon and honey to soothe the stomach. Another great tea is chamomile tea, which has antioxidant properties, can reduce bloating, and helps cleanse the stomach. It also is

considered a sleep aid. We've already discussed the benefits of mint tea earlier. You can always seek medical attention in case the symptoms worsen or if you experience stomach pain, allergies, food intolerance, diarrhea, and vomiting, which can indicate a severe issue.

4.   **Probiotics:** Take a probiotic, eat probiotic foods, and drink kombucha. I particularly like spore-based probiotics because they only activate when they hit the pH present in the small intestine. Therefore, you don't risk the stomach acid killing the beneficial bacteria. Please don't buy the cheapest; invest in probiotics that have the science to prove they can colonize in the gut. Probiotics support the gut microbiota balance and reduce the risk of infections and autoimmune diseases.

5.   **Digestive enzymes:** Enzymes are particularly beneficial as we age and in our adolescent years because chewing can be compromised at these times, and so can enzyme production in later years. Enzymes help break down the food even before it gets to the small intestine, which gives more surface area for your enzymes to break down the food further.

6. **Daily Health:** We have reviewed many practices, such as monitoring your stool, exercise, relaxation and managing stress, sleep, and more. All of these healthy habits help the health of the gut. As we work on the other pillars of longevity, the gut health pillar will also improve.

LEAVE A 1-CLICK REVIEW!

Customer reviews

⭐⭐⭐⭐⭐ 5 out of 5

141 global ratings

5 star		97%
4 star		3%
3 star		0%
2 star		0%
1 star		0%

˅ How customer reviews and ratings work

Review this product

Share your thoughts with other customers

Write a customer review

I would be incredibly thankful if you could take just 60 seconds to write a brief review on Amazon, even if it's just a few sentences!

7

THE NON-NEGOTIABLES

And Next Steps

First, let's discuss what's non-negotiable for good health. If any one of these items is off, they must become a priority because there is no amount of compensation that you can make to correct their imbalance.

- Sleep: We have dedicated an entire chapter to explaining the benefits of sleep. I am sure you will begin to prioritize sleep and treat it as the most effective medication for your health that's required daily.

- Water Intake: Too many of the body's vital systems require water to operate effectively. The cardiovascular, circulatory, urinary, and lymphatic systems must have water to work efficiently. Your gut cannot be healthy without it. Your body must have an appropriate amount of water; recognizing that fact is your first step to adjusting your water immediately.

- Daily Bowel Movements: Your bowel movements are a leading indicator of gut health, and gut health is a non-negotiable for longevity. It must be an effective selective barrier system allowing nutrients and preventing toxins into the body. Monitor your bowel movements.

- Regulation of Blood Sugar Levels: The body cannot have hormonal balance with blood sugar swings. Following a diet plan that reduces or eliminates high-glycemic foods is a start. Both the Mediterranean and MMD work beautifully in blood sugar regulation, but if you're not ready to take that step, begin eliminating refined carbohydrates and reducing high glycemic load foods.

Next Steps

Now that you have all the information necessary to live the most extended, healthiest life possible, knowing how to implement these strategies into your lifestyle can be overwhelming. The idea is to balance all the pillars because they work together. You need to be consistent and focus on improved progress and not perfection. It is a life plan; you don't need to rush through it but give attention to all the pillars and improve them regularly.

Changing overnight and attempting to implement the ideal recommendations immediately is unrealistic for those who aren't healthy. When I was first diagnosed with Crohn's Disease, the dietary changes of no dairy, beef, gluten, or preserved and processed foods were about impossible, but baby steps allowed me to implement them a little at a time. To get you started, I will give you simple and actionable steps for each pillar you can start today.

I'll have suggestions for each pillar broken down into four steps.

- Step 1 - Beginner

- Step 2 - Intermediate
- Step 3 - Advanced
- Step 4 - Master

Look at each step, and if you are already accomplishing one of them, then make your goal the next step. If you're not accomplishing step 1, that is where you should begin.

Pillar One: Sleep Your Way to Health

Step One

- Prioritize your sleep. Treat sleep as a doctor's prescription.

- Manage your time and set aside a minimum of seven hours of sleep every night, which usually means a minimum of eight hours in bed.

- Eat your final meal three hours before bed and make it a light meal containing no more calories than a third of your BMR.

- Avoid alcohol and caffeine a few hours before bedtime.

- Try to be consistent but don't give up when you fail one day. Keep at it, and the body will adjust over time.

Step Two

- Implement everything in step one

- Establish consistent sleep and wake times. Sleep and wake up at the same time every day, even on weekends.

- If you're waking up without an alarm with only seven hours of sleep, you can continue with only seven hours. However, if you rely upon your alarm to wake, then increase your time in bed until an alarm isn't necessary.

Step Three

- Implement everything in steps one and two.

- Create a good sleep environment. Create a dark environment and maintain the right temperature. Your body temperature should drop when you're asleep, so the temperature in your room should be lower than what you're used to during waking hours by about 3 degrees.

Step Four

- Implement every step above

- Begin a bedtime routine. Do relaxing activities every night before sleep, such as taking a warm bath, listening to relaxing music, meditating, or reading a book. Do the same activities every evening.

- Remove all electronic gadgets in your bedroom and eliminate their use within 30 minutes of your bedtime.

Pillar Two: Eat to Live

Step One

- Drink adequate water.

- Implement a 12/12 time-restricted eating schedule. In this plan, you restrict eating to twelve hours daily. You can eat between 8 am and 8 pm, for example.

- Switch your white foods to whole grains, such as rice and bread.

- Read the labels, eliminate all trans fats, and reduce saturated fats.

Step Two

- Drink adequate water.

- Implement a 16/8 time-restricted eating schedule. In this plan, you restrict eating to eight hours daily. For example, you can eat between 12 pm and 8 pm or 7 am and 3 pm.

- Switch your white foods to whole grains, such as rice and bread.

- Read the labels, eliminate all trans fats, and reduce saturated fats as much as possible. Increase your unsaturated fats.

Step Three

- Drink adequate water.

- Implement a 16/8 time-restricted eating schedule. In this plan, you restrict eating to eight hours daily. For example, you can eat between 12 pm and 8 pm or 7 am and 3 pm.

- Follow the ideal meal plan for the Mediterranean Diet.

  o Eat more fruits, vegetables, whole grains, legumes, fish, other seafood, and natural herbs and spices.

  o Increase healthy fats such as avocado, nuts, seeds, olive, and avocado oil.

  o In moderation (only a couple of times weekly, if ever), eat eggs, chicken, turkey, cheese, milk, and yogurt.

  o Avoid consuming red meat, added sugars, processed foods such as sausage, and refined grains.

  o The diet also allows moderate red wine and limits all other alcohol. You can take a glass of wine with dinner.

Step Four

- Drink adequate water.

- Implement a 16/8 time-restricted eating schedule. In this plan, you restrict eating to eight hours daily. For example, you can eat between 12 pm and 8 pm or 7 am and 3 pm.

- Implement a bi-annual CERF to obtain the benefits of long-term fasting as recommended in chapter three, *Eat to Live.*

- Remain on the Mediterranean Diet or transition to the MMD.

  o Eat more fruits, vegetables, whole grains, legumes, fish, other seafood, and natural herbs and spices.

  o Increase healthy fats such as avocado, nuts, seeds, olive, and avocado oil.

  o In moderation (only a couple of times weekly, if ever), eat egg whites, low-fat poultry, low-fat and lactose-free milk, and dairy.

  o Eliminate consuming red meat, added sugars, processed foods such as sausage, and refined grains.

- The diet also allows moderate red wine and limits all other alcohol. You can take a glass of wine with dinner.

Pillar Three: Exercise

Step One: Total time invested each week is 64 minutes.

- Stability: Complete the balancing exercises noted in Chapter 4 for five minutes twice weekly.

- Strength Training: 1 15-minute session weekly. Alternate upper body and lower body each week.

- Zone 2 Cardio: 2 15-minute sessions getting your heart rate to 60-70% of its max.

- Zone 5 Anaerobic: 1-minute high-intensity training (HIT), 2 minutes recovery, three repetitions, once weekly.

Step Two: Total time invested each week is two hours and 20 minutes.

- Stability: Complete the balancing exercises noted in Chapter 4 for 10-minutes, a minimum of twice weekly.

- Strength Training: 2 20-minute sessions weekly. Alternate upper body and lower body.

- Zone 2 Cardio: 2 30-minute sessions getting your heart rate to 60-70% of its max.

- Zone 5 Anaerobic: 2 minutes high-intensity training (HIT), 3 minutes recovery, four repetitions.

Step Three: Total time invested each week is 3 hours and 40 minutes.

- Stability: one hour of yoga or Pilates class weekly.

- Strength Training: 2 25-minute sessions weekly. One upper body and the other lower body.

- Zone 2 Cardio: 3 30-minute sessions weekly.

- Zone 5 Cardio: 3-minute HIT, 3 minutes recovery, five repetitions. Once weekly.

Step Four: Total time invested each week is 5 hours and 40 minutes weekly.

- Stability: One hour of yoga or Pilates class weekly.

- Strength Training: 2 30-minute sessions weekly. One upper body and the other lower body.

- Zone 2 Cardio: 4 or more 45-minute sessions

- Zone 5 Anaerobic: 4-minute HIT, 4 minutes recovery, five repetitions.

Pillar Four:
Relaxation and Your State of Mind

- **Step One**5-10 minutes of autogenic relaxation or meditation twice weekly.

- **Step Two:** 5-10 minutes of autogenic relaxation or meditation twice per week and a 10–15-minute creative visualization session once weekly.

- **Step Three:** Three 8–15-minute meditation sessions weekly with at least one session incorporating creative visualization.

- **Step Four:** 10-15 minutes of meditation once or twice daily with at least two weekly sessions intended for physical relaxation and at least one session incorporating creative visualization.

Pillar Five: Elimination and Detoxification

These steps correlate with the healthy diet prescribed in the *Eat to Live* next step recommendations. You cannot improve the gut by jumping to step 4 if you don't also commit to improving your diet. Improve your food intake to improve and maintain your gut health.

If you have significant symptoms, I recommend working with a practitioner to test for a leaky gut, SIBO, and SIFO, and recondition the gut if necessary instead of easing into a healthy gut, as the steps below suggest.

- **Step One:**
  - Fix any stomach acid deficiencies described in chapter 6.

- **Step Two:**

- Fix any stomach acid deficiencies described in chapter 6.

- Add a probiotic supplement, preferably spore-based, to maintain gut health or add probiotic foods.

- Add digestive enzymes to your daily routine if you are over 40 years old. All supplements aren't created equal, so we recommend getting advice from a practitioner. I've also included recommendations you can find at the conclusion of this book.

- **Step Three:**

  - Fix any stomach acid deficiencies described in chapter 6.

  - Add a probiotic supplement, preferably spore-based, to maintain gut health. And add probiotic foods.

  - Add digestive enzymes to your daily routine. All supplements aren't created equal, so we recommend getting advice from a practitioner. I've also included recommendations you can find at the conclusion of this book.

- o Use the Food, Mood, Poop Journal to track sensitivities and eliminate foods that cause bloating, gas, and fatigue.

- **Step Four:**

  - o Fix any stomach acid deficiencies described in chapter 6.

  - o Add a probiotic supplement, preferably spore-based, to maintain gut health. And add probiotic foods.

  - o Add digestive enzymes to your daily routine. All supplements aren't created equal, so we recommend getting advice from a practitioner. I've also included recommendations you can find at the conclusion of this book.

o Use the Food, Mood, Poop Journal to track sensitivities and eliminate foods that cause bloating, gas, and fatigue.

o Implement a biyearly preventive gut reconditioning protocol (work with a qualified practitioner).

CONCLUSION

Throughout *Longevity Secrets*, we have explored how lifestyle change can improve the quality of your life, reduce gut problems, and even reverse chronic diseases such as type two diabetes. The human body is one extensive connected system that works concurrently. High-stress levels affect the gut, and an imbalance of the gut microbiome can cause anxiety and depression. The good news is that when you address the five pillars of health, you take care of all the body systems.

Most diseases can be prevented by a good diet, regular activity, sleep, relaxation, and proper digestive health. The longevity secrets are the pathway to better memory, an active lifestyle, and being pain-free, or significantly reducing pain, for the rest of your life. Start to implement this plan by setting up your environment for success.

Don't depend only on your willpower. Clear your pantry from unhealthy refined, and processed foods and stock up on healthy foods. Keep your electronics outside your bedroom and incorporate more activities into your lifestyle. The brain chooses the easy path, so make it easy for yourself to follow the health plan in this book. If you keep away from unhealthy junk, you increase your chances of success. Your lifestyle determines 90% of your health outcomes, and you are in charge. Take the driver's seat, and don't let yourself down. You can live long without pain, memory loss, or prescription medication.

I have shared concepts that have changed my life, and my patients and family's lives. I have used these concepts to help my patients have medication-free and pain-free lives. I have seen these practices reverse type two diabetes, high cholesterol, GERD, and hypertension and eliminate chronic pain, anxiety, depression, and leaky gut by addressing the root cause of these diseases.

Your body knows how to treat itself; you need to give your body what it needs, and it will do the rest. You now have the knowledge and the step-by-step guide. How will you use your new knowledge? It may be difficult at first to change habits that you have been doing for years. Behavior change is not an automatic switch on and off system. It takes time. Be patient with yourself. But don't delay. Start today!

The steps in this book apply to everyone, no matter their health or fitness level. Make small changes in each pillar until they become part of your lifestyle. Take small incremental steps and build your way up. Balance all the five pillars because they are related. Balance and consistency are critical to this plan's success.

Now that you have all the tools go out there and use them. Share this knowledge with your family and friends and support each other to take the plunge to a long and healthy life. You only have one life. Take care of it.

ABOUT THE AUTHOR

Life has a way of leading us to our fate, and Tammy Gallagher's life was no exception. She became overweight in her twenties, developed high blood pressure and high cholesterol, and was diagnosed with Crohn's disease in her late forties. She spent most of her adult life in the residential development industry but left the industry in her early 50s as she realized she was trading her health for money. She was operating on autopilot and wasn't happy, so she sought to change.

Tammy learned that 'giving up' is never an option, and she finally returned to college in her fifties to get the degree she wanted. Tammy is a functional nutrition and lifestyle practitioner and author; best yet, she received her health and life back. She now shares the wisdom gained from her experience and education with others as a means of encouragement and support.

In 2018 Tammy decided that she wanted to give back more to the world than she had been able to do by continuing her journey toward mastering a healthy body and mind. She opened Ballantyne Weight Loss Center to help others achieve health as well.

As a businesswoman, Tammy understands that changing one's life requires vision, determination, and perseverance. This book aims to provide people with inspiration and advice on how to live a healthier lifestyle and add years to their lives.

LEAVE A 1-CLICK

REVIEW!

Customer reviews

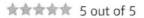 5 out of 5

141 global ratings

5 star		97%
4 star		3%
3 star		0%
2 star		0%
1 star		0%

⌄ How customer reviews and ratings work

Review this product

Share your thoughts with other customers

Write a customer review

I would be incredibly thankful if you could take just 60 seconds to write a brief review on Amazon, even if it's just a few sentences!

OTHER BOOKS YOU'LL LOVE

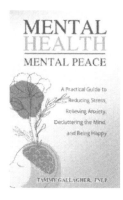

Mental Health – Mental Peace
amazon.com/dp/B0BJTJ2HRQ

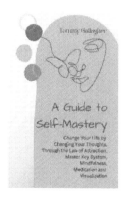

A Guide to Self-Mastery
amazon.com/dp/B0BL52NNPP

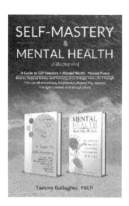

Self-Mastery & Mental Health
amazon.com/dp/B0BM3PFL3F

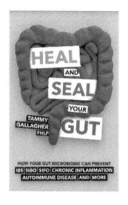

Heal and Seal Your Gut
Coming Soon!

Just for You!

A FREE GIFT FOR OUR READERS

Get my free eBook on sweeteners...the good, the bad and the ugly. Which sweeteners to avoid and which provide health benefits.

Visit *www.tamgall.com/sweeteners-ebook*

RECOMMENDATIONS

The products recommended throughout *Longevity Secrets* are below. To view all supplements recommended by Tammy Gallagher, you can create an account here:

https://gchiropractic.gethealthy.store/customer/account/create/

1. Alta Water in-home filtration system: www.altawater.com/tamgall
2. Prolon: Fasting Mimicking Diet
    a. Original: https://gchiropractic.gethealthy.store/catalog/product/view/id/2295/s/prolon/
    b. Soup Variety 2: https://gchiropractic.gethealthy.store/catalog/product/view/id/10281/s/prolon-soup-variety-2/
    c. Three Month Supply: https://gchiropractic.gethealthy.store/catalog/product/view/id/5425/s/prolon-3-month-supply/
3. Digestive Enzymes: https://gchiropractic.gethealthy.store/digestive-enzymes-ultra-with-betaine-hcl-90-capsules.html
4. Probiotics:

a. https://gchiropractic.gethealthy.store/catalog/product/view/id/5090/s/megasporebiotic/

b. https://gchiropractic.gethealthy.store/probiotic-50b.html

5. Apple Cider Vinegar Tablets: https://gchiropractic.gethealthy.store/apple-cider-vinegar.html

6. Multivitamin: https://gchiropractic.gethealthy.store/o-n-e-multivitamin.html

7. Fiber:

a. https://gchiropractic.gethealthy.store/g-i-fortify-capsules.html

b. https://gchiropractic.gethealthy.store/catalog/product/view/id/3856/s/purelean-fiber/

8. Gut Restoration Products:

a. https://gchiropractic.gethealthy.store/catalog/product/view/id/10683/s/epiintegrity-powder-6-oz/

b. https://gchiropractic.gethealthy.store/o-n-e-omega.html

c. https://gchiropractic.gethealthy.store/catalog/product/view/id/3856/s/purelean-fiber/

d. https://gchiropractic.gethealthy.store/catalog/product/view/id/5090/s/megasporebiotic/

9. Mental Health – Mental Peace: A Practical Guide to Reducing Stress, Relieving Anxiety, Decluttering the Mind and Being Happy: https://www.amazon.com/dp/B0BHTT9264

10. A Guide to Self-Mastery: Change Your Life by Changing Your Thoughts Through the Law of Attraction, Master Key System, Mindfulness, Meditation and Visualization: https://www.amazon.com/dp/B0BL418P63

11. Self-Mastery – Mental Health: How to Relieve Stress and Anxiety, and Change Your Life Through the Law of Attraction, Meditation, Master Key System, Mindfulness and Visualization. 2-Books-in-1: https://www.amazon.com/dp/B0BLV4SP9V

12. Kombucha Recipe: http://mycrohnslife.com/

ILLUSTRATION PERMISSIONS

Figures were provided courtesy of the author except for the following.

Fig 1: Modified from https://unsplash.com/photos/feKxV48FZVM

Fig 2: Modified from https://unsplash.com/photos/tEVGmMaPFXk

Fig 3: Modified from https://www.pexels.com/photo/an-elderly-couple-doing-yoga-8939944/

Fig 4: Modified from https://www.pexels.com/photo/a-fit-couple-in-a-runner-s-lunge-pose-7500322/

Fig 5: Modified from https://www.pexels.com/photo/an-elderly-man-exercising-8899512/

Fig 6: Modified from https://www.pexels.com/photo/woman-exercising-bear-body-of-water-1300526/

REFERENCES

1. Watson, N. F., Badr, M. S., Belenky, G., Bliwise, D. L., Buxton, O. M., Buysse, D., Dinges, D. F., Gangwisch, J., Grandner, M. A., Kushida, C., Malhotra, R. K., Martin, J. L., Patel, S. R., Quan, S. F., & Tasali, E. (2015). Recommended Amount of Sleep for a Healthy Adult: A Joint Consensus Statement of the American Academy of Sleep Medicine and Sleep Research Society. *Sleep*, *38*(6), 843–844. https://doi.org/10.5665/sleep.4716

2. Center for Disease Control and Prevention. (2021, March 12). *Do You Get Enough Sleep? | CDC*. Retrieved October 9, 2022, from https://www.cdc.gov/chronicdisease/resources/infographic/sleep.htm

3. *Sleep in America® Polls*. (2022, September 19). National Sleep Foundation. Retrieved October 9, 2022, from https://www.thensf.org/sleep-in-america-polls/

4. Pacheco, D. (2022, August 10). *Why Do We Need Sleep?* Sleep Foundation. Retrieved October 9, 2022, from https://www.sleepfoundation.org/how-sleep-works/why-do-we-need-sleep

5. Itani, O., Jike, M., Watanabe, N., & Kaneita, Y. (2017). Short sleep duration and health outcomes: a systematic review, meta-analysis, and meta-regression. *Sleep medicine, 32*, 246–256. https://doi.org/10.1016/j.sleep.2016.08.006

6. Charest, J., & Grandner, M. A. (2020). Sleep and Athletic Performance: Impacts on Physical Performance, Mental Performance, Injury Risk and Recovery, and Mental Health. *Sleep medicine clinics, 15*(1), 41–57. https://doi.org/10.1016/j.jsmc.2019.11.005

7. Nagai, M., Hoshide, S., & Kario, K. (2010). Sleep duration as a risk factor for cardiovascular disease- a review of the recent literature. *Current cardiology reviews, 6*(1), 54–61. https://doi.org/10.2174/157340310790231635

8. *How Does Sleep Affect Your Heart Health? | cdc.gov.* (2021, January 4). Centers for Disease Control and Prevention. https://www.cdc.gov/bloodpressure/sleep.htm

9. Brum, M., Dantas Filho, F. F., Schnorr, C. C., Bertoletti, O. A., Bottega, G. B., & da Costa Rodrigues, T. (2020). Night shift work, short sleep and obesity. *Diabetology & metabolic syndrome, 12*, 13. https://doi.org/10.1186/s13098-020-0524-9

10. Chattu, V. K., Chattu, S. K., Burman, D., Spence, D. W., & Pandi-Perumal, S. R. (2019). The Interlinked Rising Epidemic of Insufficient Sleep and Diabetes Mellitus. *Healthcare (Basel, Switzerland), 7*(1), 37. https://doi.org/10.3390/healthcare7010037

11. Oh, C. M., Kim, H. Y., Na, H. K., Cho, K. H., & Chu, M. K. (2019). The Effect of Anxiety and Depression on Sleep Quality of

Individuals With High Risk for Insomnia: A Population-Based Study. *Frontiers in neurology*, *10*, 849. https://doi.org/10.3389/fneur.2019.00849

12. Eugene, A. R., & Masiak, J. (2015). The Neuroprotective Aspects of Sleep. *MEDtube science*, *3*(1), 35–40.

13. Beattie, L., Kyle, S. D., Espie, C. A., & Biello, S. M. (2015). Social interactions, emotion and sleep: A systematic review and research agenda. *Sleep medicine reviews*, *24*, 83–100. https://doi.org/10.1016/j.smrv.2014.12.005

14. *How poor sleep can ruin your social life*. (2018, August 22). University of California. https://www.universityofcalifornia.edu/news/how-poor-sleep-can-ruin-your-social-life

15. Irwin, M. R., Olmstead, R., & Carroll, J. E. (2016). Sleep Disturbance, Sleep Duration, and Inflammation: A Systematic Review and Meta-Analysis of Cohort Studies and Experimental Sleep Deprivation. *Biological psychiatry*, *80*(1), 40–52. https://doi.org/10.1016/j.biopsych.2015.05.014

16. Harvard Health. (2022, January 11). *How sleep deprivation can cause inflammation*. Retrieved October 9, 2022, from https://www.health.harvard.edu/sleep/how-sleep-deprivation-can-cause-inflammation

17. Mawer, R. M. (2020, February 28). *17 Proven Tips to Sleep Better at Night*. Healthline. Retrieved October 9, 2022, from https://www.healthline.com/nutrition/17-tips-to-sleep-better

18. *Sleep tips: 6 steps to better sleep*. (2022, May 7). Mayo Clinic. Retrieved October 9, 2022, from

https://www.mayoclinic.org/healthy-lifestyle/adult-health/in-depth/sleep/art-20048379

19. *The importance of hydration.* (2018, June 22). News. Retrieved October 9, 2022, from https://www.hsph.harvard.edu/news/hsph-in-the-news/the-importance-of-hydration/

20. Panel on Dietary Reference Intakes for Electrolytes and Water; Standing Committee on the Scientific Evaluation of Dietary Reference Intakes; Food and Nutrition Board; Institute of Medicine. (n.d.). *Read "Dietary Reference Intakes for Water, Potassium, Sodium, Chloride, and Sulfate" at NAP.edu.* Retrieved October 9, 2022, from https://nap.nationalacademies.org/read/10925/chapter/6

21. Bodybuilding.com, & Writer, C. (2021, July 27). *BMR Calculator: Learn Your Basal Metabolic Rate for Weight Loss.* Bodybuilding.com. Retrieved October 9, 2022, from https://www.bodybuilding.com/fun/bmr_calculator.htm

22. *Basal Energy Expenditure.* (n.d.). Retrieved October 9, 2022, from http://www-users.med.cornell.edu/%7Espon/picu/calc/beecalc.htm

23. *What to Know About Intermittent Fasting for Women After 50.* (2021, March 22). WebMD. Retrieved October 9, 2022, from https://www.webmd.com/healthy-aging/what-to-know-about-intermittent-fasting-for-women-after-50

27. *Foods to Keep You Healthy as You Age.* (2009, December 7). WebMD. Retrieved October 9, 2022, from

https://www.webmd.com/healthy-aging/features/longevity-foods

29. Shiffer, E. (2022, January 31). *A Complete Guide To The Mediterranean Diet And How It Can Help You Lose Weight.* Women's Health. Retrieved October 9, 2022, from *Benefits of Physical Activity.* (2022, June 16). Centers for Disease Control and Prevention. Retrieved October 9, 2022, from https://www.cdc.gov/physicalactivity/basics/pa-health/

30. *Benefits of Physical Activity.* (2022, June 16). Centers for Disease Control and Prevention. Retrieved October 9, 2022, from https://www.cdc.gov/physicalactivity/basics/pa-health/

31. *Long-term benefits of regular exercise.* (2017, April 4). YMCA of the North. Retrieved October 9, 2022, from https://www.ymcanorth.org/blog/2017/04/04/5991/long_term_benefits_of_regular_exercise

32. Mishra, N. (2011, July 1). *Exercise beyond menopause: Dos and Don'ts Mishra N, Mishra V N, Devanshi - J Mid-life Health.* Retrieved October 9, 2022, from https://www.jmidlifehealth.org/article.asp?issn=0976-7800;year=2011;volume=2;issue=2;spage=51;epage=56;aulast=Mishra

33. Flanagan, B. (2022, June 17). *Framework for exercise.* Peter Attia. Retrieved October 9, 2022, from https://peterattiamd.com/framework-for-exercise/

34. Attia, P. (2022, September 1). *#206 - Exercising for longevity: strength, stability, zone 2, zone 5, and more.* Peter Attia.

Retrieved October 9, 2022, from https://peterattiamd.com/exercising-for-longevity/

35. WebMD Editorial Contributors. (2020, November 16). *Best Balance Exercises for Seniors*. WebMD. Retrieved October 9, 2022, from https://www.webmd.com/healthy-aging/best-balance-exercises-for-seniors

36. LeWine, H. E., MD. (2013, November 1). *Balance training seems to prevent falls, injuries in seniors*. Harvard Health. Retrieved October 9, 2022, from https://www.health.harvard.edu/blog/balance-training-seems-to-prevent-falls-injuries-in-seniors-201310316825

37. Skolnik, B. . S. P. W. H. (2022, May 13). *7 Reasons Why Strength Training Is Key to a Long Life*. AARP. Retrieved October 9, 2022, from https://www.aarp.org/health/healthy-living/info-2022/strength-training-and-longevity.html

38. Andrejs. (2022, August 2). *Heart Rate Training Zones – Complete Guide To Endurance Gains*. The Athlete Blog. Retrieved October 9, 2022, from https://theathleteblog.com/heart-rate-training-zones/

39. Attia, P. (2022a, September 1). *#92 - AMA #12: Strategies for longevity (which don't require a doctor)*. Peter Attia. Retrieved October 9, 2022, from https://peterattiamd.com/ama12/

40. INTEGRIS Health. (n.d.). *Why It's Important to Allow Yourself to Rest*. Retrieved October 9, 2022, from https://integrisok.com/resources/on-your-health/2021/april/why-its-important-to-allow-yourself-to-rest

41. *Relaxation techniques: Try these steps to reduce stress.* (2022, April 28). Mayo Clinic. Retrieved October 9, 2022, from https://www.mayoclinic.org/healthy-lifestyle/stress-management/in-depth/relaxation-technique/art-20045368

42. Staff, M. (2022, September 2). *How to Meditate.* Mindful. Retrieved October 9, 2022, from https://www.mindful.org/how-to-meditate/

43. INTEGRIS Health. (n.d.-a). *Meditation 101: How to do it and why it makes us feel better.* Retrieved October 9, 2022, from https://integrisok.com/resources/on-your-health/2020/november/benefits-of-meditation

44. Hoshaw, C. (2021, June 9). *How Long Should You Meditate to Get the Benefits? Here's What the Science Says.* Healthline. Retrieved October 9, 2022, from https://www.healthline.com/health/mind-body/how-long-should-you-meditate-to-get-the-benefits-heres-what-the-science-says

45. *Physical Relaxation Techniques: Deep Breathing, PMR, and Centering.* (n.d.). Mind Tools. Retrieved October 9, 2022, from https://www.mindtools.com/pages/article/newTCS_05.htm

46. *High optimism linked with longer life and living past 90 in women across racial, ethnic groups.* (2022, June 8). News. Retrieved October 9, 2022, from https://www.hsph.harvard.edu/news/press-releases/optimism-longevity-women/

47. Marillea Yu Nd. (2022, March 7). *Detoxification & Elimination: A Quick Overview.* The Clara Clinic. https://theclaraclinic.com/blog-home/detoxification-and-elimination-a-quick-overview

48. Precision Nutrition. (n.d.). *6 reasons you should care about your poop health.* Retrieved October 25, 2022, from https://www.precisionnutrition.com/poop-health

49. Ballantyne Weight Loss Center. (2021, July 28). *Leaky Gut Repair - Ballantyne Weight Loss Center.* Ballantyne Weight Loss Center - Fast Long Term Weight Loss. https://ballantyneweightloss.com/leaky-gut-repair/

50. Xu, H., Liu, M., Cao, J., Li, X., Fan, D., Xia, Y., Lu, X., Li, J., Ju, D., & Zhao, H. (2018). The Dynamic Interplay between the Gut Microbiota and Autoimmune Diseases. *Journal of Immunology Research,* 2019. https://doi.org/10.1155/2019/7546047

51. Andrea Nakayama. (February 2020). Full Body Systems. Functional Nutrition Alliance.

52. *Hypochlorhydria (Low Stomach Acid): Symptoms, Tests, Treatment.* (n.d.). Cleveland Clinic. Retrieved October 25, 2022, from https://my.clevelandclinic.org/health/diseases/23392-hypochlorhydria

53. Sissons, C. (2022, July 29). *8 ways to improve digestion.* https://www.medicalnewstoday.com/articles/325822

54. Harvard Health. (2016, February 19). *Preserve your muscle mass.* Retrieved October 16, 2022, from https://www.health.harvard.edu/staying-healthy/preserve-your-muscle-mass

55. Mariotti, A. (2015, June 17). *The effects of chronic stress on health: new insights into the molecular mechanisms of brain–body communication.* Future Science. Retrieved October 20, 2022, from https://www.future-science.com/doi/full/10.4155/fso.15.21

56. National Sleep Foundation. (2015, February 2). *National Sleep Foundation Recommends New Sleep Times* [Press release]. https://els-jbs-prod-cdn.jbs.elsevierhealth.com/pb/assets/raw/Health%20Advance/journals/sleh/NSF_press_release_on_new_sleep_durations_2-2-15-1424372967217.pdf

57. *Can daylight saving time hurt the heart? Prepare now for spring.* (2021, August 16). www.heart.org. Retrieved October 21, 2022, from https://www.heart.org/en/news/2018/10/26/can-daylight-saving-time-hurt-the-heart-prepare-now-for-spring

58. Altomare, R., Cacciabaudo, F., Palumbo, V. D., Gioviale, M. C., Bellavia, M., Tomasello, G., & Lo Monte, A. I. (2013, March 1). *The Mediterranean Diet: A History of Health.* National Library of Medicine - PubMed. https://www.ncbi.nlm.nih.gov/pmc/articles/PMC3684452/

59. Attia, P. (2022, September 1). *How does VO2 max correlate with longevity?* Peter Attia. https://peterattiamd.com/how-does-vo2-max-correlate-with-longevity/

61. Newgen, H. (2022, January 4). *Most Likely Cause of Your Visceral Fat, Say Experts.* Eat This Not That. Retrieved October 21, 2022, from https://www.eatthis.com/news-likely-causes-of-your-visceral-fat-say-experts/

62. *Visceral Fat: What It is & How to Get Rid of It.* (n.d.). Cleveland Clinic. Retrieved October 21, 2022, from https://my.clevelandclinic.org/health/diseases/24147-visceral-fat

63. Leffler, S. (2021, September 7). *The #1 Cause of Belly Fat, Says Dietitian.* Eat This Not That. Retrieved October 21, 2022, from https://www.eatthis.com/one-cause-of-belly-fat-dietitian/

64. Crosby, J. (2017, August 10). *Leaky Gut and Metabolic Syndrome.* Crosby Chiropractic & Acupuncture Centre. Retrieved October 21, 2022, from https://www.crosbychiropractic.com/leaky-gut-and-metabolic-syndrome/

65. Albosta, M. (2021, February 3). *Intermittent fasting: is there a role in the treatment of diabetes? A review of the literature and guide for primary care physicians - Clinical Diabetes and Endocrinology.* BioMed Central. Retrieved October 21, 2022, from https://clindiabetesendo.biomedcentral.com/articles/10.1186/s40842-020-00116-1

66. Patterson, R. E., Laughlin, G. A., Sears, D. D., LaCroix, A. Z., Marinac, C., Gallo, L. C., Hartman, S. J., Natarajan, L., Senger, C. M., Martinez, M. W., & Villasenor, A. (2015, April 6). *INTERMITTENT FASTING AND HUMAN METABOLIC HEALTH.* National Library of Medicine - PubMed. Retrieved October 21, 2022, from https://www.ncbi.nlm.nih.gov/pmc/articles/PMC4516560/

67. *Does intermittent fasting impact mental disorders? A systematic review with meta-analysis.* (n.d.). Taylor & Francis. Retrieved October 21, 2022, from https://www.tandfonline.com/doi/abs/10.1080/10408398.2022.2088687

68. Gudden, J. (n.d.). *The Effects of Intermittent Fasting on Brain and Cognitive Function.* MDPI. Retrieved October 21, 2022, from https://www.mdpi.com/2072-6643/13/9/3166

69. Cleveland Clinic. (2022a, January 18). *VO2 Max: How To Measure and Improve It.* https://health.clevelandclinic.org/what-is-vo2-max-and-how-to-calculate-it/

70. Universal, P. (2022, June 18). *Exercise is Better than Medicines and Cutting Out Smoking – The Best Exercises for Longevity with Peter Attia.* Parasuniversal. https://www.parasuniversal.com/2022/06/exercise-beats-drugs-and-even-stopping-smoking-the-best-exercises-for-longevity-with-peter-attia/

71. Sorriento, D., Vaia, E. D., & Iaccarino, G. (2020). Physical Exercise: A Novel Tool to Protect Mitochondrial Health.

Frontiers in Physiology, 12. https://doi.org/10.3389/fphys.2021.660068

72. *Pelvic Floor Muscles: Anatomy, Function & Conditions*. (n.d.). Cleveland Clinic. Retrieved October 25, 2022, from https://my.clevelandclinic.org/health/body/22729-pelvic-floor-muscles

73. Milanovic, Z., Sporis, G., & Weston, M. (2015, October). *Effectiveness of High-Intensity Interval Training (HIT) and Continuous Endurance Training for VO2max Improvements: A Systematic Review and Meta-Analysis of Controlled Trials*. National Library of Medicine - PubMed. https://pubmed.ncbi.nlm.nih.gov/26243014/

74. Taylor, K., & Jones, E. B. (2022, October 3). *Adult Dehydration*. National Library of Medicine - PubMed. https://www.ncbi.nlm.nih.gov/books/NBK555956/

75. Nesto, R. W. (2004). Obesity: A Major Component of the Metabolic Syndrome. *Texas Heart Institute Journal, 32*(3), 387-389. https://doi.org/https://www.ncbi.nlm.nih.gov/pmc/articles/PMC1336716/

76. Cleveland Clinic. (2022, March 3). *Intermittent Fasting: How It Works and 4 Types Explained*. https://health.clevelandclinic.org/intermittent-fasting-4-different-types-explained/

77. Lawler, M., & Kennedy, K. R. (2022, May 31). *12 Possible Health Benefits of Intermittent Fasting*. EverydayHealth.com.

https://www.everydayhealth.com/diet-nutrition/possible-intermittent-fasting-benefits/

78. *Carbohydrates*. (n.d.). Retrieved October 24, 2022, from https://medlineplus.gov/carbohydrates.html

80. Venn, B. J., & Green, T. J. (2007, December). *Glycemic index and glycemic load: measurement issues and their effect on diet-disease relationships.* National Library of Medicine - PubMed. https://pubmed.ncbi.nlm.nih.gov/17992183/

81. Dorais, S. (2021). *The Effectiveness of a Centering Meditation Intervention on College Stress and Mindfulness: A Randomized Controlled Trial.* Frontiers. https://www.frontiersin.org/articles/10.3389/fpsyg.2021.720824/full

82. Choi, I. Y., Piccio, L., Childress, P., Bollman, B., Chosh, A., Brandhorst, S., Cross, A. H., Morgan, T. E., Wei, M., Paul, F., Suarez, J., Michalsen, A., Bock, M., & Longo, V. D. (2016, June 7). *Diet mimicking fasting promotes regeneration and reduces autoimmunity and multiple sclerosis symptoms.* National Library of Medicine - PubMed. https://www.ncbi.nlm.nih.gov/pmc/articles/PMC4899145/

83. de Toledo, F. W., Grundler, F., Sirtori, C. R., & Ruscica, M. (2020, June 10). *Unravelling the health effects of fasting: a long road from obesity treatment to healthy life span increase and improved cognition.* National Library of Medicine - PubMed. https://pubmed.ncbi.nlm.nih.gov/32519900/

84. Sadeghian, M., Hosseini, S. A., Javid, A. Z., Angali, K. A., & Mashkournia, A. (2021, January 9). *Effect of Fasting-Mimicking*

Diet or Continuous Energy Restriction on Weight Loss, Body Composition, and Appetite-Regulating Hormones Among Metabolically Healthy Women with Obesity: a Randomized Controlled, Parallel Trial. National Library of Medicine - PubMed. https://pubmed.ncbi.nlm.nih.gov/33420673/

85. Fasting Mimicking Technology. (2021, September 22). L-Nutra. https://l-nutra.com/fasting-mimicking-technology/

GET FREE EBOOKS

If you'd like EARLY and FREE e-books written

by Tammy Gallagher or published by

TamGall Publishing, sign up here:

tamgall.com/book-reviewers

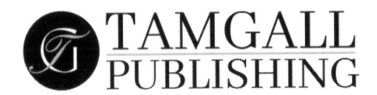

This Page is Left Intentionally Blank

Made in the USA
Coppell, TX
06 February 2023

12213611R00133